Praise for *Androgen Deprivation Therapy*

"Androgen deprivation therapy (ADT) is a life-changing event, leaving many men feeling as if they have washed up on a deserted island with no one to talk to. And that is largely true, because unless a person has been through it, and most doctors have not, it is impossible to understand how the patient feels and how to help. Until now, there has been no convenient source for patients and their physicians to get the answers that they need. At last there is a comprehensive book that covers everything: side effects, diet, exercise, psychological issues, and sexual relations. And beyond helping patients understand what is going on with their body, there is encouragement and concrete, practical exercises and solutions. Every man who is a candidate for ADT needs to read this outstanding book."
—Patrick C. Walsh, MD, University Distinguished Service Professor of Urology, Johns Hopkins Medical Institutions

"A fantastic, pragmatic, well-written book. Very comprehensive."
—Derek R. Wilke, MD, Department of Radiation Oncology, Nova Scotia Cancer Centre

"This book is an incredibly valuable resource for men with prostate cancer considering androgen deprivation therapy (ADT) and for their families and friends. It will help men to understand the pros and cons of ADT treatment and give them an idea of what to expect after they start therapy. I will certainly use it in my practice and encourage other physicians to do so as well."
—David F. Penson, MD, MPH, Hamilton and Howd Chair in Urologic Oncology, Professor of Urologic Surgery and Medicine, and Director, Center for Surgical Quality and Outcomes Research, Vanderbilt University Medical Center

"Excellent, very informative, and comprehensive. *Androgen Deprivation Therapy* addresses issues sensitively and is not afraid to tackle important but often ignored topics. I would be glad to recommend it to my patients, and their partners too."
—Paul D. Abel, ChM, FRCS (Eng), FRCS (Ed), Professor and Honorary Consultant in Urology, Imperial College London

"This book is excellent and provides important information for men on androgen deprivation therapy. It is very well written in easy-to-understand language. I will be recommending it to all my patients."
—Padraig Warde, MB, ChB, BAO, FRCPC, Professor, Department of Radiation Oncology, University of Toronto

"This book, written by internationally respected prostate cancer researchers and healthcare providers, is an invaluable resource for anyone whose life is touched by androgen deprivation therapy (ADT) for prostate cancer. Patients and their loved ones will find much reassurance that their experience is normal. Beyond reassurance, this book provides them with a road map for how to frame the ADT-related physiologic and psychological changes, how to cope with the side-effects of this treatment, and how to support

each other. Healthcare providers will find tips for how to talk to patients and their loved ones about the myriad of impacts of ADT on men's quality of life. An excellent 'go-to' handbook for every patient, family member, and clinician."
—Daniela Wittmann, PhD, MSW, Assistant Professor of Urology,
University of Michigan

"As a prostate cancer patient since 1992, activist, and mentor to prostate cancer patients and their caregivers, I am well aware of the knowledge, writings, and expertise of Richard Wassersug. Richard and his coauthors, Drs. Walker and Robinson, have dedicated much of their lives to a deep study of this insidious men's disease. In this book, Wassersug and colleagues present a wealth of information on hormone therapy. It is covered in a manner that is easily understood to ease the worry and concern for men that often follows being told, *'You have prostate cancer!'*"
—Charles (Chuck) Maack—Founder of the Prostate Advocate
(http://www.theprostateadvocate.com)

"This comprehensive guide to living and loving while on ADT should be required reading for all men prescribed this class of drugs. From the physical to the emotional and sexual side effects, this self-help book covers all the information men and their partners need."
—Anne Katz, PhD, RN, FAAN, Clinical Nurse Specialist and Certified Sexuality
Counselor

"All treatments for prostate cancer affect quality of life. This book introduces us to the potential side effects of ADT. We are then given compassionate guidance in how to adjust to those changes. As a scientist and prostate cancer survivor, I am acutely aware of the limited availability of clinical and scientific knowledge to describe the consequences of prostate cancer treatments. This book fills part of that gap by effectively lifting the 'veil' off ADT and providing a readable resource for patients considering ADT."
—Stephen Porges, PhD, Health Science Researcher and Prostate Cancer Survivor, Distinguished University Scientist, Kinsey Institute, Indiana University, Bloomington Indiana, and Professor, Department of Psychiatry, University of North Carolina

"This book should be standard reading for men and their partners prior to starting ADT. By reading and discussing the book together, couples can avoid many of the physical and psychological pitfalls that may affect couples."
—David and Dana Kababik, Prostate Cancer Survivor and Wife/Founder of
HisProstateCancer.com

"When I first read this amazing book, I have to admit that I was quite surprised. I expected to read just another book about hormone therapy (ADT) for men with prostate cancer, but this was much more.

The book offers the most open, no holds barred, honest, and thorough presentation that I have read about ADT and its side effects. It goes beyond just offering information and provides solutions as well as exercises for those who want to take advantage of them to improve their life while on ADT. This is especially true of the sections discussing intimate relationships between partners.

It is written in an easy to understand, logical progression that will enlighten both the less experienced as well as those of us who have used ADT. It is a must read for both the man undergoing or thinking of using ADT as well as his partner."

—Joel Nowak, MA, MSW, Prostate Cancer Survivor, Advocate, and
CEO of CancerABCs™ (www.cancerabcs.org)

"The first edition of *Androgen Deprivation Therapy: An Essential Guide for Prostate Cancer Patients and Their Loved Ones* gave the prostate cancer patient community their first detailed resource on ADT: written from a patient's perspective for other patients and their family members. And it dealt with one of the biggest problems in living on ADT, which is how you think about what is happening to you as a man when medical treatments radically suppress normal levels of the male hormone testosterone—and the effects that can have on you as an individual and on your interactions with others!

The general factors that affect life on ADT remain largely the same, but since the book was first published in 2014 there have been major changes: new drugs, new drug combinations, and changes in how older drugs are used. This new and updated second edition will again be an important and valuable resource for the vast majority of men who are faced with the need to start ADT for treatment of progressive and advanced forms of prostate cancer—whether for a few months or for the rest of their lives.

It is a book we will again recommend to patients when they ask us about issues related to life on ADT."

—E. Michael D. ("Mike") Scott, Co-Founder and President,
Prostate Cancer International

"I was delighted to read the second edition of the book. It's a great resource full of practical and useful information for men on androgen deprivation therapy (new or long-time users alike) and their caregivers. It clears up a number of myths and provides balanced and current information on coping with all aspects of hormone therapy.

The book has been updated to reflect the latest science and covers the gamut of issues from exercise to dealing with grief. There is great basic information for all patients and more detailed information for those who want to delve deeper. Many of my patients loved and learned a lot from the first book; I will be sure to recommend this edition to my patients, both young and old. It's also a lovely resource for health professionals who help men with prostate cancer, including doctors, nurses, psychologists, and others."

—Shabbir Alibhai, MSc, MD, FRCPC, Associate Professor, University of Toronto,
Senior Scientist, Toronto General Hospital Research Institute

"It was a pleasure reading this book. From a clinical perspective, this ADT manual is a holistic educational resource to help patients and their loved ones understand ADT and its associated consequences. The book provides a toolkit to optimize strategies for coping together."

—Catherine Paterson, PhD, Hon. Urology Nurse Consultant and Researcher in
Cancer Care, NHS Grampian and Robert Gordon University, Aberdeen, Scotland

"This book is a rich resource for any man receiving androgen deprivation therapy. In clear language, it addresses the most common and distressing effects of ADT on men and their partners. It is a workbook that guides men from knowledge to action, by helping them develop practical plans to maintain their physical and emotional health as well as their intimate relationships. I will be recommending this book to my patients."
—Kishore Visvanathan, MD, FRCSC, Clinical Professor (Urology),
University of Saskatchewan

ANDROGEN DEPRIVATION THERAPY

ANDROGEN DEPRIVATION THERAPY

AN ESSENTIAL GUIDE FOR PROSTATE CANCER PATIENTS AND THEIR LOVED ONES

SECOND EDITION

Richard J. Wassersug, PhD
Lauren M. Walker, PhD, R Psych
John W. Robinson, PhD, R Psych

With Contributions From
Kristen L. Currie, MA, CCRP; Kirsten C. Kukula, BSc, MD; Linette Lawlor-Savage, MSc; Andrew Matthew, PhD, C Psych; Deborah McLeod, RN, PhD; Daniel Santa Mina, CEP, PhD; Cheri Van Patten, RD, MSc; Erik Wibowo, PhD

Reviewed and endorsed by the Canadian Urological Association.

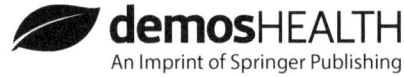

Visit our website at www.springerpub.com

ISBN: 978-0-8261-8391-0
ebook ISBN: 978-0-8261-8392-7

Acquisitions Editor: Beth Barry
Compositor: diacriTech

© 2018 by Richard J. Wassersug, Lauren M. Walker, and John W. Robinson
Demos Health is an imprint of Springer Publishing Company, LLC.

All rights reserved. This book is protected by copyright. No part of it may be reproduced, stored in a retrieval system, or transmitted in any form or by any means, electronic, mechanical, photocopying, recording, or otherwise, without the prior written permission of the publisher.

Medical information provided by Demos Health, in the absence of a visit with a healthcare professional, must be considered as an educational service only. This book is not designed to replace a physician's independent judgment about the appropriateness or risks of a procedure or therapy for a given patient. Our purpose is to provide you with information that will help you make your own healthcare decisions.

The information and opinions provided here are believed to be accurate and sound, based on the best judgment available to the authors, editors, and publisher, but readers who fail to consult appropriate health authorities assume the risk of injuries. The publisher is not responsible for errors or omissions. The editors and publisher welcome any reader to report to the publisher any discrepancies or inaccuracies noticed.

Library of Congress Cataloging-in-Publication Data

Names: Wassersug, Richard J. (Richard Joel), 1946- author. | Walker, Lauren M.
   (Lauren Marie), 1985- author. | Robinson, John W. (John Wellesley),
   1956- author.
Title: Androgen deprivation therapy : an essential guide for prostate cancer
   patients and their loved ones / Richard J. Wassersug, PhD,
   Lauren M. Walker, PhD, R Psych, John W. Robinson, PhD, R Psych ; with contributions
   from Kristen L. Currie, MA, CCRP, Kirsten Kukula, BSc, Linette
   Lawlor-Savage, MSc, Andrew Matthew, PhD, C Psych, Deborah McLeod, RN, PhD,
   Daniel Santa Mina, CEP, PhD, Cheri Van Patten, RD, MSc, Erik Wibowo, PhD ;
   reviewed and endorsed by the Canadian Urological Association.
Description: New York : Demos Health, [2018] | Includes bibliographical
   references and index.
Identifiers: LCCN 2018012467| ISBN 9780826183910 | ISBN 9780826183927 (ebook)
Subjects: LCSH: Prostate—Cancer—Hormone therapy. |
   Antiandrogens—Therapeutic use. | Prostate—Cancer—Popular works.
Classification: LCC RC280.P7 W37 2018 | DDC 616.99/463—dc23 LC record available at
   https://lccn.loc.gov/2018012467

Contact us to receive discount rates on bulk purchases.
We can also customize our books to meet your needs.
For more information please contact: sales@springerpub.com

Printed in the United States of America.

This book is dedicated to all of the men, and their partners, who have taught us what life is like on androgen deprivation therapy.

CONTENTS

Foreword by Paul F. Schellhammer, MD, FACS xi
*Preface by Richard J. Wassersug, Lauren M. Walker, and
John W. Robinson* xiii
Introduction xvii
   Before You Begin xviii
   Will Reading This Book Make Me More or Less Anxious? xx
   I Have Never Read a Manual Before—Why Start Now? xxi
   How to Read This Book xxiii
   What Are Your Values? xxiii
   Where to Go for Further Information xxiv
   Moving Forward: Questions for Discussion xxiv

1. Androgen Deprivation Therapy 1
   What Is ADT? 1
   Testosterone and DHT 9
   Moving Forward: Questions for Discussion 13

2. Physical Side Effects 15
   Hot Flashes 15
   Medications 17
   Counseling 20
   Activity: Abdominal Breathing 20
   Activity: Hot Flash Diary 21
   Weaker Bones 22
   Weight Gain and Muscle Loss 24
   Diabetes 25
   Metabolic Syndrome and Cardiovascular Risk 25
   Anemia and Fatigue 27
   Breast Growth 28
   Genital Shrinkage 30

Loss of Body Hair...31
Other Possible Side Effects..31
Activity: Pros/Cons Table...33
Activity: Action Plan...34
Activity: Goal Setting and Confidence................................35
Activity: Side Effects Self-Assessment...............................36
Physical Side Effects: Essentials....................................38
Moving Forward: Questions for Discussion............................39

3. Exercise..41
Exercising Safely..42
Warm-Up Exercises...43
Aerobic Exercises..44
Resistance Training..46
Keeping Your Bones Healthy..47
Yoga and Tai Chi..48
Cool Down..49
Making the Decision to Exercise....................................49
Activity: Pros/Cons Table...50
Activity: Matching Meaning and Change
    Using Self-Statements..52
Preparing to Successfully Begin Exercising...........................53
Activity: Action Plan...54
Activity: Goal Setting and Confidence................................55
Maintaining Your Motivation..57
Activity: Identifying and Overcoming Barriers
    to Starting and Maintaining an Exercise Program................58
Exercise: Essentials..59
Moving Forward: Questions for Discussion............................60

4. Healthy Eating..63
Reading Food Labels...64
Fats...64
Protein..66
Carbohydrates...68
Determining Your Current BMI......................................69
Estimating Your Nutritional Needs...................................70
Omega-3 Fatty Acids...71
Omega-3 Fatty Acid Supplements...................................71
Omega-6 Fatty Acids...72
Soy...73
Vitamin D...74
How Do I Get Enough Vitamin D?...................................75
Calcium...76

	Phytonutrients	78
	Polyphenols	78
	Punicalagin and Ellagic Acid	78
	Lycopene	79
	Activity: Pros/Cons Table	80
	Activity: Action Plan	81
	Activity: Goal Setting and Confidence	81
	Healthy Eating: Essentials	82
	Moving Forward: Questions for Discussion	82
5.	**Effects on Psychological Well-Being**	**85**
	Emotional Distress	86
	Emotional Expression	87
	Activity: Self-Assessment—Screening for Emotional Distress	87
	Depression	89
	Anxiety	90
	Activity: Progressive Muscle Relaxation	91
	Activity: Mindfulness Meditation	93
	Instructions	93
	Further Developing Your Mindfulness Practice	94
	Fatigue	94
	Grief	95
	Cognition	96
	Activity: Pros/Cons Table	98
	Activity: Action Plan	99
	Activity: Goal Setting and Confidence	100
	Effects on Psychological Well-Being: Essentials	101
	Moving Forward: Questions for Discussion	102
6.	**Effects on Intimate Relationships and Sexuality**	**105**
	ADT Lowers Libido	105
	Staying Close in Nonsexual Ways	106
	Making Time for Intimacy	108
	Dating	108
	Maintaining a Sexual Relationship	111
	Suggestions for Enjoying Sensual Pleasure With Low Libido	112
	Orgasms Without Ejaculation	116
	Sex: Beyond Intercourse	117
	Using Sexual Aids and Sex Toys	118
	Treatments for ED	121
	General Comments on Using Erectile Assistive Aids	122
	Activity: Beliefs Awareness	128
	Activity: Pros/Cons Table	129
	Activity: Action Plan	130
	Activity: Goal Setting and Confidence	132

Contents

7. Impact on Committed Relationships 137
    Potential Changes in the Relationship 138
    Differences in Coping Style 139
    Increased Self-Doubt 140
    Activity: Pros/Cons Table 141
    Activity: Action Plan 142
    Activity: Goal Setting and Confidence 143
    Impact on Committed Relationships: Essentials 144
    Moving Forward: Questions for Discussion 145

8. Unique Considerations for Gay Relationships 147
    ADT May Impact Committed Relationships for Gay Men .. 148
    Activity: Pros/Cons Table 149
    Activity: Action Plan 150
    Activity: Goal Setting and Confidence 151
    Unique Considerations for Gay Relationships: Essentials .. 152
    Moving Forward: Questions for Discussion 153

9. Conclusion: Staying Healthy 155

Appendix 157
    1. Drug Chart 158
    2. PSA Chart 159
    3. Hot Flash Diary 160
    4. Pros/Cons Table 161
    5. Action Plan 162
    6. Goal Setting and Confidence 163
    7. Side Effects Self-Assessment 164
    8. Screening for Emotional Distress Mood Questionnaire .. 166
    9. Beliefs Awareness Exercise 168

Glossary 169

Resources 173

Bibliography 181

Acknowledgments 193

Index 197

FOREWORD

I was honored when asked to write the Foreword to the second edition of *Androgen Deprivation Therapy: An Essential Guide for Prostate Cancer Patients and Their Loved Ones*. But full personal disclosure is appropriate and necessary.

I am a urologic oncologist who has focused on prostate cancer therapy for the past three decades. At age 50, I got my first prostate-specific antigen (PSA) test. It was 2.5 ng/mL—at that time (1990), that was considered normal; now, in 2018, it would be a red light warning for future prostate cancer worries. That concern materialized 10 years later when, at age 60, I had a radical prostatectomy for high-grade (Gleason score 4 + 4) disease. Since, I have slowly progressed with a rising PSA indicative of biochemical failure to castration-resistant metastatic disease, and I have received virtually every hormone manipulation available—luteinizing hormone-releasing hormone (LHRH) agonist, Avodart® (dutasteride), ketoconazole, Casodex® (bicalutamide), Xtandi® (enzalutamide), Zytiga® (abiraterone) with prednisone, and transdermal estrogen.

As is the case with many and perhaps most prostate cancer patients, I was forced to grapple with the new life that accompanied androgen deprivation therapy (ADT). Recognize, that as a urologic oncologist I had the advantage of a flying head start. Still, I would have benefited immensely from the information (the text, charts, video resources, discussion questions, and references) provided in this book.

Virtually every prostate cancer patient's story starts with a suspicious PSA and/or digital rectal exam followed by a biopsy, which is often followed by bone scan and CT scan imaging. Then the hard work begins. The diagnosis of prostate cancer presents a number of challenges unique to the world of malignancy. No other cancers have such a wide spectrum of primary therapies. First, should there even be immediate therapy? If active surveillance is not a consideration, should treatment be surgical and, if so, by what approach (open prostatectomy, robotic prostatectomy, perineal prostatectomy with limited or extended lymph node dissection)? Should treatment be delivered by radiation and, if so, by what method—external beam via 3-D conformal, intensity modulated radiation therapy (IMRT), proton therapy, or seed implantation (i.e., brachytherapy), alone, or in combination with external beam? Should treatment be thermal and, if so, by heating with high-intensity focused ultrasound (HIFU) or freezing with cryoablation? There is regrettably no single best treatment; each patient's situation and disease state is different. If it were clear what is the best primary treatment, this broad menu of possibilities would long ago have fallen by the wayside, making way for "the best." Clearly, when it comes to selected treatment(s) for prostate cancer, education and counseling are critically important. Fortunately, for the vast majority of prostate cancer cases, the disease progresses slowly enough to allow time for education, counseling, and discussion with other specialists.

Enter another very important therapeutic factor not mentioned in the preceding paragraph, namely ADT or hormone therapy. ADT can be a very important companion, immediate or delayed, to the treatments already listed. I use the word *companion* because ADT will travel with other therapies and also will travel with the patient for periods of time that exceed the duration of the other therapies. Indeed, it may be lifelong.

Furthermore, even after ADT has achieved its desired therapeutic effect and been discontinued, the changes it brings on can linger. In focusing on decisions regarding primary therapies such as surgery or radiation, to use a common phrase, the oxygen is sucked out of the room, and ADT runs the risk of receiving marginal attention. This must be avoided. The most certain way of avoiding this error is by having a thorough resource that supplements and expands upon patient–physician discussions and decisions. This book is that resource. It is a comprehensive manual that details what to expect and, equally as important, how to address, modify, and adjust to the side effects of ADT. The immediate perceived side effects of ADT may be dramatic while other changes in body systems (i.e., in muscle, bone, sexual, metabolic, and cognitive function) may be more subtle. Both require attention and countermeasures to relieve and minimize.

For the first edition of this book published in 2014, I wrote "It was only when I began my personal journey with androgen deprivation therapy that I was able to appreciate the profound impact this treatment has on daily life. Even with my real life experience with ADT, accumulated over decades, I know I cannot, within the limits of one or even several office visits, begin to prepare and educate patients for the new reality. I could not even do that for myself! If only a complete user-friendly manual existed. Now it does." For patients beginning ADT, who thankfully have the promise of improved survival, this statement holds true more than ever.

Paul F. Schellhammer, MD, FACS
Past President of the American Urological Association
Professor, Department of Urology
Eastern Virginia Medical School
Norfolk, Virginia

PREFACE

Androgen deprivation therapy (ADT, often called hormone therapy) is a common treatment for prostate cancer, but it has a wide range of side effects. This book presents techniques to minimize the burden from those side effects. Most physicians who prescribe ADT typically warn patients about the most serious effects, but many have admitted to us that they do not have the time to discuss all of the side effects that a patient might experience. Nor do they typically have the time to cover all options for dealing with those side effects. As one oncologist told us, speaking for all physicians who treat patients with ADT, "In spite of our best efforts to educate patients and their partners about ADT, we often still feel we are not doing enough."

Our goal with this book is to fill in what may not get covered in the clinic when a physician tells a patient, "I recommend that you start on hormone therapy."

How did we come to be so interested in this topic?

Some 20 years ago Richard Wassersug was diagnosed with prostate cancer, when he was in his early 50s. His specific interest in ADT began 2 years later, when he was offered ADT as a treatment for his cancer that had failed to be controlled by surgery and subsequent radiation therapy. At the time, Richard was a professor of Anatomy and Neurobiology in Dalhousie University's Medical School in Halifax, Canada. As a researcher, he was so surprised by how ADT affected how he felt and thought—and the limited information he could find on how to deal with that—that he began investigating the psychosocial impact of ADT.

To sort out physiological reality from placebo effects, he started by looking at how rodents in the laboratory responded to androgen deprivation. Erik Wibowo joined him in this research, first as a PhD student and later as his postdoctoral fellow. Richard also began communicating with other prostate cancer patients and their partners from around the world via online chat groups. This advanced his knowledge about what others were going through with ADT. It also helped him acquire skills in communicating with others about how to maintain a good quality of life when the patient is on ADT.

John Robinson is a clinical psychologist who started working with prostate cancer patients in the 1980s at the Tom Baker Cancer Centre in Calgary, Canada. Back then it was common for men on ADT to suffer in silence, hesitant to admit that they were suffering. They did not want to be thought of as weak and did not want others to know how their cancer treatment made them feel emasculated. Even when their physicians inquired about how they were doing, many men minimized their distress, often dismissing it as "no big deal."

This conspiracy of silence meant that most men suffered alone. Initially, John saw few referrals for men on ADT in his clinical practice. However, as an increasing number of men, like Richard, spoke publicly about their life on ADT, more men followed. Knowing that they were not alone made it easier to acknowledge what they were going through and to request support. Today, John's practice is full of men and their partners, who want information on how to live well while on ADT.

Lauren Walker began working with men on ADT in 2007 as a student under John's supervision. For her master's thesis she studied the impact of ADT on couples. She continued on as a PhD student evaluating a draft edition of this book. Like John, Lauren is now a clinical psychologist and researcher working with cancer patients and their partners at the Tom Baker Cancer Centre and the University of Calgary.

Lauren has a passion for helping underserved populations, which aligns well with her investigation of the unique needs of men on ADT. As a clinician, researcher, and educator, Lauren now facilitates classes as part of our ADT educational initiatives for men and their partners, and champions access to such services for patients not just in Calgary, but across all of Canada.

One focus of our collaborative research is to increase the understanding about the challenges posed by ADT. A key starting point occurred a decade ago, when we established the ADT Working Group. This brought together about 20 researchers and clinicians from the United States and Canada to develop guidelines for supporting men on ADT and their partners. The first edition of this book, published in 2014, arose from our initiative to improve the knowledge of patients, partners, physicians, and other healthcare providers about how to manage ADT side effects.

As background to the book, we investigated what clinicians felt patients starting on ADT needed to know and also what patients knew about the side effects of ADT. In many cases, our research demonstrated that patients did not know enough about the treatment to be prepared to manage ADT side effects. That was a stimulus for us to develop educational initiatives for patients, partners, and healthcare professionals to help them recognize and manage those changes brought on by ADT.

This book goes well beyond the standard conversations prostate cancer patients might have with their doctors and other healthcare providers. It is structured as a workbook, which means that it includes not just information but also exercises, which you can go through at your own pace. The book need not be read straight through; instead, each chapter is more or less freestanding.

The book covers not only the physical side effects of ADT but the psychological side effects that can alter how one feels and how one interacts with loved ones. Importantly, the book recognizes that ADT impacts not just patients, but also their partners and others close to them. For the book to be most effective for couples, we encourage both patients and partners to read the book and to explore together the questions and exercises at the end of each chapter.

We are delighted by the success of the first edition of this book. In this new edition, we have expanded the text in response to feedback from patients, who asked for more information on the drugs used for ADT and the context for administering them. We have also expanded the discussion of side effects and their management, which is the primary focus of the book. The Resource and Bibliography sections at the end of the book are greatly expanded too, with an added new chapter on the psychological impact of ADT on gay men.

Whether you are about to start ADT, live with someone about to start on ADT, or have been on ADT for several years, you should be able to find here evidence-based strategies for maintaining a good quality of life while on this treatment.

Richard J. Wassersug, PhD
Vancouver, British Columbia

Lauren M. Walker, PhD, R Psych
Calgary, Alberta

John W. Robinson, PhD, R Psych
Calgary, Alberta

INTRODUCTION

This book is designed to help prostate cancer patients and their loved ones learn about and deal with the side effects of androgen deprivation therapy (ADT), commonly referred to as hormone therapy. You may have already received some information from your physician, nurse, or pharmacist about why ADT is being prescribed and the common side effects of this treatment. This book will provide you with more information about ADT and prepare you for what you might experience from ADT. Not all patients experience every side effect, and side effect severity varies from patient to patient. We hope that by using this book you will be better able to adjust to ADT, cope with its impact on your life, and manage the side effects that you experience.

Most patients tell us that they prefer to know about all possible side effects ahead of time, rather than be surprised by any side effects, even when there is only a small chance of experiencing them.

You may find that some strategies provided here seem like a good fit for you, while others do not. Use what works for you. It may be helpful to read the book at the start of treatment, or shortly before, and then again some months later. Material that may not have seemed relevant initially may become more so over time when you start experiencing certain side effects.

There is also some information here for the loved ones of men on ADT. Some sections are appropriate for all loved ones; others are specifically for sexual partners.

Openly discussing the side effects can make it easier to adapt overall and may help you learn ways of managing the side effects so you have a better quality of life. It is important to discuss your concerns with your healthcare providers before you start ADT *and* during treatment.

- It is important to maintain open communication with your partner, family, and friends, as well as with your doctor and nurse.
- Keep your doctor updated about how you feel about the treatment and how you are dealing with the side effects.
- There is help available if you are struggling. Please do not wait until you are overwhelmed to ask for help.

Before You Begin

We believe the value of this book is enhanced when patients and loved ones discuss ADT-related issues *together*. Questions at the end of each section are designed to help you think about how this information applies to you and to facilitate communication with your loved ones. Some questions specifically address couples; others are appropriate for individuals, or for patients who are dating or hope to date in the future. Even if you do not have a person you feel you can talk to about your concerns, we hope you will still think over these questions and answer them for your own benefit.

> **If you are currently in an intimate relationship, we recommend that you and your partner work to maintain a strong, supportive bond with each other. This requires open and honest communication. If you are not in a relationship, you may consider asking a close friend or family member to discuss with you some of the topics that are raised in this book.**

Here are some questions to consider before you begin. Try to answer all of them. There are no right or wrong answers. Taking time to reflect upon the questions, and writing down your answers, may be helpful. Use the space provided.

Questions:

- Who can I talk to about my concerns and about this book?
- What does it mean to me to be on ADT?
- What do I already know about ADT?
- What questions do I have about ADT?
- Which potential side effects are of most concern to me?
- How comfortable am I in talking about sex with my partner, a close friend, or with my physician?

If you are in a relationship, some specific questions for couples include:

- How will our relationship change as a result of ADT?
- How might any changes affect my partner?
- Which side effects have the potential to change our relationship?
- What do we value most about our relationship?
- How comfortable are we talking to each other about sensitive issues, such as sex?
- How well do we communicate on a day-to-day basis?
- What areas of our communication could be improved?

NOTES:

_____

_____

_____

_____

_____

_____

_____

_____

_____

_____

_____

_____

_____

Will Reading This Book Make Me More or Less Anxious?

Some individuals are very laid back about gathering information on their illness and its management. Psychologists refer to such people as *blunters*. They generally take a relaxed approach to healthcare. They may seem less distressed, but they may miss out on critical information. Blunters may want only the essential information about ADT and find this book to be too detailed.

Monitors, on the other hand, are individuals who like to learn the details of a condition and all of the options available to them, including treatments and side effects—but they do tend to worry more. Monitors may want even more detail than what they will find here.

One style is not any better than the other. If you find that you and your partner have different styles, you can enlist each other's help. Knowing your tendencies and your partner's tendencies may help both of you deal with the challenges to come.

If you are a blunter, and the idea of reading the whole book is unappealing to you, here are some suggestions:

- Select certain parts to read by looking at the Table of Contents or Index. Skim through the chapters, reading the topics that interest you the most.
- Read the questions at the end of each chapter.
- Ask someone to read the book and point out to you the sections that are most relevant.

If you are a monitor, you may appreciate how detailed this book is, but you may also find yourself getting anxious reading some parts. If you do, look for the reassuring messages throughout, and remember:

- Not all patients experience all side effects.
- There are many things that you can do to keep your body, mind, and relationship strong and healthy.
- There are steps you can take to manage the impact of ADT on you and your life.

I Have Never Read a Manual Before—Why Start Now?

When we hand patients a copy of this book, they often say to us, "I have never read a manual before—why start now?" To help answer that question, here is a story drawn from our interactions with one particular patient. We hope his perspective encourages you to make the most of this book, instead of just skimming it.

When my doctor said I should start hormone therapy, he told me I might have a few side effects, like hot flashes, gaining a few pounds, and I might lose interest in sex. He suggested I take vitamin D and calcium to keep my bones strong. That didn't sound too bad.

He also gave me this book and said it might help me deal with the side effects. I wasn't sure I needed to read it. I'd seen my wife deal with hot flashes, and we mostly just joked about it. I always ate healthy and walked the dog so I didn't think I had to worry about my weight. I'd been using Viagra since my surgery so we had already gotten used to not having sex like we used to. And I knew my marriage was solid. We've been together for 30 years—what is there that we couldn't handle? I'd dealt with lots of adversity in the past and overcome it, so I had every confidence that I would adapt this time too. Besides, I'd never read a manual before—I've always been able to figure things out on my own. Why start now?

I figured I would take things a day at a time, but I was surprised when the changes slowly crept up on me. I tried to joke about the hot flashes, but I was really embarrassed when I was in a business meeting and got all red in the face and broke out in a sweat. One day, when I got out of the shower, I really looked at myself in the mirror. Somehow, I had developed a beer belly. I'd always taken pride in being in good shape and here I'd put on 15 pounds, without even noticing.

That day, I looked at my body and saw that my penis had shrunk and my testicles too! I was angry that no one told me that my genitals would shrink after beginning on ADT. I started to feel really down about myself and my ability to satisfy my partner. Even though my mood started to tank, I told myself I needed to suck it up and not make a big deal of it.

I did my best to ignore these changes, but I started to notice that my wife seemed unhappy. I asked her what was wrong. She was very reluctant to say anything at first. I had to encourage her to say what was on her mind. She then started to point out how I had changed and how our relationship had changed. She said I had withdrawn from her both physically and emotionally. She told me she understood that I might not have the desire to have sex; what

I didn't notice was that I had stopped regularly touching her. My kisses had become mechanical.

She feared we had become more like brother and sister than husband and wife. I had become grumpy and sometimes was short with her. I seemed tired and unenthusiastic about life. She went on to say that she was saddened by the changes and felt lonely, but was reluctant to bring this all up because she knew it wasn't my fault. She was patiently waiting, hoping that we would just adapt to these changes with time.

After my wife told me how she felt, I realized that I needed to do something. I didn't know what to do, so I started by calling my doctor's office. We got a referral to a counselor willing to talk with us. When my wife and I went to see the counselor, he asked if I'd read this book. I had to admit that I'd only glanced at it and hadn't really read it. In fact, I had forgotten all about it. I promised I would dig it out and read it before our next meeting.

I was surprised to learn in the book that there are things I could try to control the hot flashes. I learned about the importance of physical activity in keeping my weight under control and stopping the loss of muscle mass. I realized that there were things I could have been doing to help prevent myself from being in this situation.

Also, reading the material and doing the exercises with my wife was actually really helpful. It helped us to understand what was happening between us and what other couples on hormone therapy did to keep their relationship strong. I was surprised to learn how some couples even continue to enjoy sexual activity. Reading this book turned my life around. In hindsight, I think it could have helped to prevent a lot of suffering for both my wife and me.

I don't know why I was so reluctant to read it. I guess I had assumed that these things were not going to happen to me. I told one of my engineering friends that I wished I'd read the book back when I started on hormone therapy like my doctor had suggested. He asked, "Have you ever heard the expression RTFM?" I hadn't, so I went online and searched the term. Do you know what it stands for? If you don't know what it means, and won't be offended by strong language, you might want to do an online search too.

Perhaps this book should come with that recommendation, "RTFM," in bold letters. It may be crass, but it's advice best taken. My wife now makes a point of teasing me about it, and I have a good laugh when I make this recommendation to other men starting on this treatment.

Although ADT is given only to the patient, the effects of ADT can produce physical and emotional changes in the patient that may indirectly affect his loved ones. The goal of this book is to help both patients and loved ones recognize and adapt to the side effects of ADT.

How to Read This Book

This book is structured as a workbook, with the chapters having many specific questions to be explored and exercises intended for both patients and loved ones. Many of the questions are meant to stimulate discussion. Just reading the book may benefit both patients and their loved ones, but the greatest benefit can come from both patients and those close to them discussing together their answers to the questions we ask in the book. There is some redundancy between chapters, which reflects the fact that the chapters were written to be largely freestanding. For example, some terms may be redefined, and specific activities designed to help you make changes in your life are repeated at the end of each chapter. This was done because we recognize that the needs of individuals vary greatly and not everyone will need to read every chapter of this book in detail.

You will notice that Chapter 7 is titled "Impact on Committed Relationships" and that Chapter 8 is titled "Unique Considerations for Gay Relationships," yet some of the content in Chapter 7 is still relevant for gay men. However, Chapter 7 does not adequately capture the complexity of nonheterosexual relationships. There is also a section in the middle of Chapter 7 called "Effects on Intimate Relationships and Sexuality" that is devoted to dating; this is likely irrelevant for those who are already in committed relationships. Please do not feel that the only way to read this book is from front to back. You can be selective on the chapters you elect to read, as they are largely independent from each other. We encourage you to pick and choose the chapters that are most relevant to you and also to your loved ones.

What Are Your Values?

One activity that might help you decide which chapters of the book you would like to focus on is a *values clarification exercise*. In the past few years, our team has developed an educational program to help patients on ADT and their partners manage the side effects of ADT, and in that program we often ask patients (and their partners) to reflect on the areas of their lives that they consider priorities. Priority areas may include and are not limited to physical ability, energy, education and learning, physical appearance, relationships, sexuality, healthy living, and so on.

For example, one patient might say, "My family life is particularly important to me and I want to maintain good relationships, and have the energy to invest in those relationships." For him, protecting his mood and working to counteract fatigue might be key areas to focus on as he reads through the book. Another patient might say, "My physical fitness and stamina are most important to me, as I like to hike and engage in a variety of recreational and leisure activities." For him, learning more about how to manage muscle mass loss, weight gain, and metabolic syndrome might be the most important areas of the book. Still another patient might say, "My career is important to me and maintaining my mental capacity, organization, and skills is essential to me being good at my job"; therefore, focusing in on the cognitive and psychological chapter of the book might be essential for him.

Where to Go for Further Information

Associated with this book is our website, www.LIFEonADT.com. This site provides additional information on ADT. For instance, there are tables there that give the names of the common drugs used for ADT in most English speaking countries outside of North America. On the LIFEonADT homepage there are three short introductory videos about how our ADT Educational Program and this book might help you in adapting to ADT. On subsequent pages, there are a series of videos (the "Videos" link can be found in the left-hand navigation pane) that introduce brief discussions with real patients and partners about specific topics covered in the book (e.g., hot flashes, physical fitness, adapting to sexual changes such as reduced sexual desire or erectile dysfunction). There are also videos on making healthy lifestyle changes that teach you how to complete the various activities that can be found at the end of each chapter of the book, including one of a patient completing the aforementioned *values clarification exercise*. You will also find a section at the back of this book containing information on additional resources as well as a glossary of medical terms.

Moving Forward: Questions for Discussion

Following are questions that should help you to reflect on the material in this section and how it may affect you. Try to answer each question.

- How do you react to illness in general—are you more of a monitor or a blunter?
- What have you already heard from either healthcare professionals or others about the side effects of ADT?
- Do you have specific questions that you would like to have answered about the form of ADT that you have been offered and the side effects of the treatment?
- Have you discussed with your physician how long you might need to be on ADT and whether you are a candidate for intermittent ADT?

NOTES:

ANDROGEN DEPRIVATION THERAPY

1

ANDROGEN DEPRIVATION THERAPY

As a patient, you are about to begin treatment with drugs that reduce the amount of male hormones, called androgens, in your body. The main androgens are **testosterone**[1] and **dihydrotestosterone (DHT)**. This treatment, while commonly called hormone therapy, is more properly called **androgen deprivation therapy (ADT)**.

What Is ADT?

ADT is effective in controlling prostate cancer and treating most of the symptoms associated with prostate cancer. ADT works by reducing testosterone (produced in the **testicles**), the main **hormone** that stimulates the growth of prostate cancer cells. An additional small amount of testosterone is normally produced in the body by the adrenal glands. Suppressing the amount of testosterone in the body can slow the spread of your prostate cancer and significantly reduce the symptoms associated with the disease. Many men benefit, often for years, from ADT.

Testosterone affects many other tissues in the body in addition to the prostate gland, and men on ADT typically experience changes and side effects related to the lack of testosterone. Many patients and their loved ones readily accept the side effects of ADT in return for a life-prolonging treatment and recognize the trade-off between some quality of life for quantity of life. Other patients and their loved ones struggle to adjust to the side effects. We focus here on how you can maintain a good quality of life while on ADT.

[1]Technical terms are in bold in the text the first time they are used and are defined in the Glossary.

ADT causes prostate cancer tumors to shrink, but may not kill them. It is thus understood as a treatment that is therapeutic, but usually not curative. Since it can significantly extend one's life while minimizing cancer symptoms, patients on ADT can view their cancer as a chronic disease similar to high blood pressure or diabetes. For these conditions, medications are taken to manage, rather than to cure, the illness. With good management of a chronic illness, even when primary treatment has failed, a patient can still expect to live a good, long life. Many patients on ADT can realistically expect to live long enough to see further improvements in treatment. A cure may still be found. Starting on ADT does not mean that one will die of prostate cancer. In fact, most prostate cancer patients do not die from prostate cancer itself, but from other disease.

Good management of chronic diseases means changing one's lifestyle. The same can be said for living well on ADT.

How Does ADT Work?

Androgen deprivation is commonly achieved by administering drugs (see the tables on page 4) in the form of a simple injection. These injections contain a pellet that slowly releases a synthetic hormone which blocks a chemical signal from the brain—specifically from the **pituitary gland** located at the base of the brain—that normally tells the testicles to produce testosterone. The most common drugs used for ADT are called **LHRH agonists** or **GnRH agonists**. LHRH stands for luteinizing hormone-releasing hormone and GnRH stands for gonadotropin-releasing hormone, but the different names refer to the same hormone. A different class of drugs called **GnRH antagonists** (or **LHRH antagonists**) can also shut down that signal to the testicles, with similar side effects. In addition, the different drugs may be sold under different names in countries outside of North America. For the alternative names in major English-speaking countries, see the tables at www.LIFEonADT.com.

With the injections, you may also be prescribed oral medications called **antiandrogens** (see the table in the following discussion). These drugs work quite differently than the injectable LHRH agonists and antagonists. They block the ability of testosterone (and other androgens) to attach to the cancer cells, the process which normally stimulates the cancer cells to grow. Some cells may then die, but others unfortunately may survive and mutate such that they are then able to grow even without testosterone. Thus, like the LHRH drugs, antiandrogens alone are not considered curative in the long run, but they can help control the cancer.

Commonly, patients who are prescribed an LHRH agonist are advised to start taking an oral antiandrogen 2 to 3 weeks before getting their first LHRH agonist injection. For some patients, it may be beneficial to stay on the antiandrogen long-term, but for others it may not be necessary. This is a decision that should be made in consult with your physician. When an LHRH drug and an antiandrogen are taken together, they are often referred to as *combined androgen blockade* (CAB), *total androgen blockade* (TAB), or *maximum androgen blockade* (MAB). Some patients also refer to this combination as **ADT2**.

The table at the top of page 4 lists commonly prescribed LHRH drugs and their relevant information.

The second table on page 4, "Antiandrogen Drugs Commonly Used to Treat Prostate Cancer," lists commonly used antiandrogens that may be prescribed to work in conjunction with injectable medications to achieve CAB, or given to patients short-term for a few weeks before starting on an LHRH agonist. In some geographic regions, antiandrogen drugs are used alone at a high dose as a form of ADT, but this is not common in North America.

There are other drugs recently introduced into clinical practice that also impact the hormonal environment in the body, including enzalutamide (Xtandi®), apalutamide (Erleada®), and abiraterone (Zytiga®). These drugs are playing an increasing role in managing advanced prostate cancer.

Enzalutamide and the new drug apalutamide are new and particularly potent oral antiandrogens. Abiraterone is another oral drug that blocks testosterone production. Abiraterone blocks testosterone production or synthesis, not only from the testicles but also from the adrenal glands, by blocking the enzyme that normally converts a precursor molecule into testosterone. Drugs like abiraterone are so effective in reducing testosterone that they have been referred to in the recent medical literature as causing "androgen annihilation" rather than androgen deprivation. There are many promising studies looking at early use of these two compounds as alternatives to the more established LHRH agonist drugs, or in combination with them.

Enzalutamide, apalutamide, and abiraterone have their own side effects, and these can intensify some of the side effects of the LHRH drugs. Also, because abiraterone not only blocks testosterone production in the adrenal glands, but other compounds synthesized there, abiraterone has to be taken with a synthetic steroid drug, called prednisone. The prednisone compensates for the loss of those other essential compounds necessary for other bodily functions.

Although not commonly used in North America as a first-line hormone therapy, female hormones called **estrogens** can also be used to suppress testosterone. These can be either natural (e.g., **estradiol**) or synthetic (e.g., **diethylstilbestrol [DES]**) compounds. At high concentrations, like the LHRH drugs, they can reduce the hormonal signals from the brain to the testicles to produce testosterone. The oral forms of these drugs have been associated with an elevated risk of blood clot formation and are now rarely used in North America and Europe. However, if taken nonorally, such as through the skin (e.g., via a patch or gels), the risk for clots is much lower. Research is underway to see if nonoral estrogens are as effective in cancer control, with fewer bothersome side effects, than the LHRH drugs. As discussed in Chapter 2, estrogenic compounds can help reduce some of the side effects of the LHRH drugs.

LHRH Drugs Commonly Used to Treat Prostate Cancer

Generic Name	Trade Name	How Is the Drug Given?[a]	How Often Is the Drug Given?
Leuprolide	Lupron® Eligard®	Intramuscular injection Subcutaneous injection	Every 1, 3, 4, or 6 months[b] Every 1, 3, 4, or 6 months[b]
Goserelin	Zoladex®	Subcutaneous injection	Every month or every 3 months[b]
Triptorelin	Trelstar®	Intramuscular injection	Every 1, 3, or 6 months[b]
Buserelin	Suprefact®	Subcutaneous injection Nasal spray	Every 3 months Daily
Degarelix[c]	Firmagon®	Subcutaneous injection	Two initial injections and then monthly injections

LHRH, luteinizing hormone-releasing hormone.
[a] Subcutaneous injections are given under the skin, usually in the abdomen. Intramuscular injections are usually injected into the muscle of the buttock.
[b] Frequency of injections depends on the dose.
[c] Unlike the other drugs listed here, degarelix is an LHRH antagonist rather than an LHRH agonist.
Note: The dosage and location of injection may vary between drugs, but the long-term side effects are largely similar whether the drugs are agonists or antagonists. After the injection is administered, you may feel tenderness and/or itchiness and a small lump under the skin at the injection site.

Antiandrogen Drugs Commonly Used to Treat Prostate Cancer

Generic Name	Trade Name	How Is the Drug Given?	How Often Is the Drug Given?
Bicalutamide	Casodex®	Pill	Daily
Flutamide	Eulexin®	Pill	Three times daily
Nilutamide	Nilandron® (United States) Anandron® (Canada)	Pill Pill	Daily Daily
Enzalutamide	Xtandi® (United States)	Pill	Daily
Apalutamide	Erleada® (United States)	Pill	Daily

Androgen Synthesis Blocker Drugs Used to Treat Prostate Cancer

Generic Name	Trade Name	How Is the Drug Given?	How Often Is the Drug Given?
Abiraterone	Zytiga® (United States)	Pill	Daily

LHRH Agonists Versus Antagonists

In common English, an agonist and antagonist have opposing effects. However, because of the complicated nature of the hormonal control of the testicles, LHRH agonist and antagonist drugs end up having the same effect on androgen production. They both shut off the hormonal signal from the pituitary gland that tells the testicles to make testosterone. The testicles depend on that signal; without it, they stop making testosterone. The following paragraphs go into greater detail on the differences between an LHRH agonist and antagonist. They are presented here for those interested in such details and are not specifically related to side effect management.

The difference in the two classes of drugs relates to a hormone signal from a region in the brain called the **hypothalamus**. The hormonal control of the testicles is a two-step process. The hypothalamus sends a signal to the pituitary to make the hormone that triggers the testicles to produce testosterone. The antagonists simply shut down the signal from the hypothalamus to the pituitary.

The agonists work in a more complicated and indirect fashion, but the ultimate result is the same; that is, testosterone production from the testicles is shut down. The agonist mimics the normal signal from the hypothalamus to the pituitary. It is a strong signal that puts the pituitary into overdrive. The pituitary at first increases the signal to the testicles to make testosterone. However, after a couple weeks of this excessive exposure, the cells in the pituitary do not respond to the LHRH anymore. As a result, the pituitary stops sending a signal to the testicles to produce testosterone. And that shuts down testosterone production in the testicles.

Although in the long term, the result is the same—that is, the testicles do not get the signal from the pituitary to make testosterone, so they shut down—the patient's initial experience on these two treatments is not the same. The most commonly used agents for ADT are the agonists. Within a few days of starting therapy, a patient on these drugs experiences an initial rise in his testosterone. If you start on the drugs because of symptomatic **metastatic** disease, that initial surge of testosterone can cause those **metastases** to swell, which may cause pain. This is called "flare" and it is something to be avoided. The reason that patients initiating ADT with LHRH agonists commonly start by taking antiandrogen at the time of (or a few weeks before) their first injection is to block the testosterone produced in that initial surge from promoting the growth of tumor cells and the associated flare.

Antagonists have the advantage, over agonists, of driving down the testosterone faster and without the risk of flare. Thus, the antagonist is the drug of choice when a patient first presents for treatment with symptomatic and painful metastases. You may wonder, "Why not always just use a LHRH antagonist rather than an agonist?" Despite the fact that, with the antagonist, there is no initial rise in testosterone, no flare, and no need to precede the ADT injection with antiandrogen pills, administration of the antagonists can be a bit more difficult. As you can see from the first table on page 4, when a patient starts on a drug like degarelix, it requires two depot injections instead of one. Also degarelix is administered monthly whereas the agonists come as longer acting depots and require fewer injections. Injecting degarelix can be a bit challenging and some men report discomfort at the injection site with some swelling or redness. With either class of drugs some patients may feel a lump from the material injected, but this typically subsides in the coming days to weeks. For these reasons, the most common drugs used for testosterone suppression remain the LHRH agonists. In fact, it is not uncommon for patients who start on an antagonist for 2 or 3 months to then switch over to a more convenient agonist.

The Original ADT

In the early 1940s, a physician and research scientist, Dr. Charles Huggins, suspected that prostate cancer growth may be influenced by male hormones. He is credited with pioneering the idea that certain cancers could be hormone dependent. He then went on to prove this and for that he won the Nobel Prize in medicine in 1966. Back in the 1940s there were none of the sophisticated pharmaceuticals now used to shut down testosterone production or block androgens from attaching to cancer cells and stimulating their growth. Thus, the only way of lowering the patients' testosterone was to remove the testicles—which is called surgical **castration** or **orchiectomy**.

The language used in the prostate cancer literature still reflects the surgical origins of ADT. Advanced prostate cancer, which can no longer be controlled by androgen deprivation, is referred to as "castration resistant." In this situation, the **prostate-specific antigen (PSA)** may continue to rise despite the patient being on one or more androgen-suppressing agents. (A more detailed explanation of PSA is included toward the end of this chapter.) This is in contrast to the situation when the PSA level can be controlled by ADT, which is called "hormone sensitive." Occasionally there may be a distinction in the literature between "medical" and "surgical" castration. The former refers to suppressing testosterone with drugs and the latter to an orchiectomy.

Huggins soon began to offer his patients the synthetic estrogen DES, the first drug option for ADT, as an alternative to surgical castration. Since DES was relatively inexpensive and came in a pill form, it was perceived as less traumatic and more manageable for the patient than an orchiectomy. However, oral DES was found to have a high risk of blood clot formation. There was, thus, an effort to find safer drugs for ADT. Leuprolide was the first synthetic LHRH drug and began to replace DES for ADT in the late 1980s. Leuprolide was and remains much more expensive than DES, but has a lower risk of causing dangerous blood clots.

The pharmacological approach to ADT has been preferred over the surgical approach for the simple reason that it can be discontinued. For patients who only need short-term ADT—for example, to enhance the effectiveness of radiotherapy that is being used to treat prostate cancer that is localized or confined to the prostate gland—this pharmacological treatment makes the most sense. But for patients who have advanced disease and need continuous ADT, some arguments can be made to consider an orchiectomy. A more detailed discussion of the context for continuous versus intermittent and long-term versus short-term ADT can be found toward the end of the chapter. The majority of drugs used for ADT are expensive; thus if one is likely to be taking them for the rest of his life, an orchiectomy will be a cheaper option in the long run. Although the psychological impact of a surgical castration may be assumed to be greater than the impact of medical castration, there has been hardly any research on that topic. One study actually found that patients getting ADT drug injections were overall more anxious than those who got an orchiectomy. The difference the researchers suggested was that those patients on the LHRH drugs had the stress of repeated doctors' visits to receive their injections and more frequent PSA tests. Heightened anxiety may have been associated with waiting for test results. In contrast, the surgical patients had a single operation—a 1-day procedure—and did not require as frequent clinic visits.

Currently surgical castration for ADT remains common in parts of the world where financial resources are more limited. An orchiectomy is a credible alternative to the LHRH drugs if one has advanced prostate cancer and needs continuous testosterone suppression. Chemical and surgical ADT offer comparable cancer control. Furthermore, surgical ADT has not been shown to differ significantly in side effects or to cause greater psychological stress in the long term. Therefore, although surgical castration is the oldest form of ADT, it is still a viable option for some patients. DES is also still used in many parts of the world, primarily because it is inexpensive. Some relatively recent research in the United States has reexplored using it for ADT, but at a lower dose than what was used back in the 1960 to 1980s. This reduced dose seems to have a lower blood clot risk and may otherwise help patients, where cost is a concern, to avoid some of the more bothersome side effects of the LHRH drugs.

Physicians vary in their views of these early therapies. Some older physicians may remember prostate cancer patients who died of blood clots from oral DES. They may avoid DES altogether, and consider any estrogen compound, no matter the method of delivery, as too risky for prostate cancer patients. This assumption ignores new data suggesting that it is not the compounds but how they are administered that is the problem.

As for surgical castration, many men, whether patients or physicians, consider an orchiectomy as crude and archaic. For both patients and physicians, the language can be a problem. The word *castration* can be scary and as such people often avoid this precise terminology in favor of vague language that is potentially confusing. The best example of this is itself the term *hormone therapy*. For most other medical situations hormone therapy implies replacement of a hormone, not its removal (which is the case for ADT). Our own studies show that many people do not understand what "hormone therapy" means as a treatment for prostate cancer. As such, many patients offered "hormone therapy" may not have enough information to make an informed decision about whether or not to accept that treatment and may also be less prepared to manage ADT side effects when they emerge.

The Future of ADT

There are many remarkable and promising new changes to ADT administration. These are in part a result of newer drugs, which have been shown to extend life, but they are also a result of advances in personalized medicine. Let us look at these two factors separately.

With an increasing number of drugs available to treat prostate cancer, a couple of questions arise. First, what is the best order to use the drugs? So far, no ADT-related drug has been identified as curative, but they do show some benefit to many patients. We can now legitimately talk about not just first- and second-line ADT options, but first, second, third, and fourth ADT protocols, and so on. An enormous number of clinical trials are underway to figure out the best order to administer the growing number of treatment options available to patients on ADT. Some will prove to be better for early stage disease while others are already proving to be more effective when used later, as the disease progresses.

Second, there is lots of research exploring using approved treatments in new combinations. For example, because chemotherapy for prostate cancer has not been found to be curative and has substantial side effects, it is often reserved for treating very advanced metastatic disease. However, recently it has been shown that combining ADT with chemotherapy and using such combined treatments earlier can substantially extend life for some patients. In a similar vein, there is new evidence suggesting that combining and simultaneously administering both old and new ADT agents (such as LHRH agonists with abiraterone and prednisone) may be more beneficial than using LHRH agonists followed by abiraterone, at least for some patients. Patients can expect to see a lot of research in the coming years that explores the timing of ADT, the order of ADT treatments, and using the various treatment combinations. All of this research will take time, and the more effective the drugs are in initially controlling the cancer, the longer duration is needed for the studies to prove that they truly improve survival overall.

Overlaying all this is the issue of matching treatments to individual patients' health status and genetics, as well as the genetics of their tumors. This is within the promising area of personalized medicine and is a fast evolving field—one changing so fast that any attempt we might make to present a status report would soon be obsolete. So what does this all mean for patients starting on ADT? There are several points that patients need to consider. First, they should appreciate that ADT is not a single form of treatment, but now a raft of various treatments. All treatments have benefits and risks. As such, patients need to explore with their physicians what might be the best protocol for them to start on, and continue to ask their physicians what second- and third-line ADT protocols are available, if the first one proves less than ideal. Patients should also expect, as part of personalized medicine, that the physicians treating them will take into consideration their overall health in deciding what ADT protocol is best for them. If the patients have comorbidities—for example, diabetes, previous **cardiovascular** events, or osteoporosis—they may be directed toward one treatment over another and have not just their PSA, but also other measures of their health, monitored along the way.

Patients who live near research hospitals may be invited to participate in clinical trials that are testing the best order, timing, and combination of ADT treatments. Increasingly, patients in ADT clinical trials can expect to have their overall health and possibly their genetics (and that of their tumors) monitored. This monitoring is done through genetic data collected from the tumor or blood samples. Patients can be optimistic though, since progress has been made for several decades now, with the death rate from prostate cancer continually going down. Much of this reflects better diagnosis and treatments. Even without a cure yet found, increasingly powerful treatments that substantially extend life are now available. Advanced prostate cancer can often be controlled for long periods of time as a chronic disease. Your focus as a patient thus needs to be on managing treatment side effects in order that you and those close to you maintain a good quality of life for as long as possible.

Testosterone and DHT

Some of the testosterone in a man's body is converted to another androgen called **dihydrotestosterone** (DHT). DHT binds to receptors on prostate cells like testosterone does, and it is a more potent stimulus for the growth of prostate cancer cells.

Medications that block the conversion of testosterone to DHT, such as finasteride (Proscar®) and dutasteride (Avodart®), are often prescribed to manage symptoms related to benign enlargement of the prostate (called *benign prostatic hypertrophy* [BPH]). Both are oral medications. The benefits of these medications in managing prostate cancer are uncertain. Some patients may be prescribed these drugs to help with urinary complaints. Some clinicians and patients refer to using this drug together with LHRH agonists and antiandrogens as "triple blockade," or **ADT3**. There is no clinical evidence that ADT3 is significantly more effective at controlling prostate cancer than the LHRH drugs used alone or when combined with an antiandrogen.

What Medications Are You Taking for ADT?

The following chart can help you to track the ADT drugs that have been prescribed for you. An additional copy is available in the Appendix on page 158.

Medication	Dose and Starting Date	How Often?

How Long Will I Be on ADT?

The duration of ADT recommended to you will depend upon your situation.

Life-long ADT is prescribed in either of these two circumstances:

1. The PSA continues to rise after completion of primary treatments, such as **prostatectomy**, **brachytherapy,** or **external beam radiotherapy** and, given the patient's age and general health status, is at high risk of fatal disease if not further treated.
2. The cancer is known to have spread beyond the prostate.

Some patients are on ADT for a while, and then stop and take a "drug holiday." Cycling on and off the drug is known as *intermittent hormonal therapy*. Whether intermittent therapy is the best program for you will depend upon how well your cancer is controlled and how your PSA level behaves over time. The case for "going intermittent" is that for many patients it can limit the side effects of treatment while still maintaining good overall, long-term cancer control.

Short-term ADT is often recommended, from 6 months to 3 years, for patients with cancer confined to the prostate gland who go for some form of radiotherapy as a primary treatment. In this situation, ADT is often given for a few months prior to the start of the radiation therapy and continued throughout the radiotherapy treatment period, as well as for several months afterward. These patients may be recommended to stay on the drugs longer if their cancer appears to be more aggressive. However, newer studies suggest that ADT, when given to enhance radiotherapy, can be effective for many patients when administered for a shorter period of time, ranging from 6 to 18 months. There is an increasing amount of research showing that the benefits of using ADT to support radiotherapy varies based on the overall health of patients and how advanced their cancer is when they start radiotherapy.

What Is the PSA Test?

PSA is a protein produced by cells of the prostate gland. The **PSA test** measures the level of PSA in a man's blood. For this test, a blood sample is sent to a laboratory for analysis. PSA is present in small quantities in the blood of men with healthy prostates, but is often elevated in the presence of prostate cancer or other prostate disorders.

How Is the PSA Test Used for Men Who Have Been Treated for Prostate Cancer?

An increase in PSA in a patient who has had treatment for prostate cancer *may* be a sign of a recurrence of the disease. A single elevated PSA in a patient who has a history of prostate cancer is not a guarantee of recurrent cancer, and it is often necessary to repeat PSA testing over time to identify trends before confirming recurrence of the disease. Such recurrence is called a *biochemical relapse* or *biochemical failure* if (a) the PSA rises over time, and if (b) examination and diagnostic imaging (e.g., **CT** or bone scans) do not identify tumor deposits related to prostate cancer. If the examination or diagnostic imaging shows that there has been a spread of the cancer, it is called *metastatic disease*.

How Is the PSA Test Used When You Are on ADT?

A PSA that remains low indicates that your cancer is being controlled. If you are on intermittent therapy, ADT is stopped when the PSA drops to a very low level and remains in that range for at least a few months.

If the PSA level rises above a specific threshold, ADT is started again. How high the PSA is allowed to rise before stopping or starting back on ADT is a matter to discuss with your physician. There have not been enough large-scale, long-term studies to provide solid rules for when to stop or restart ADT. In general, the decision needs to take into consideration how to ensure that you have the best cancer control and, concurrently, the best overall quality of life.

How Good Is the PSA Test?

With rare exception, the PSA level is a good indicator of the effectiveness of treatment. Generally speaking, your PSA should be very low while on ADT, but this can vary. The PSA level itself does not predict whether or not a man will have symptoms or how long the man will live. Many men have very high PSA values (e.g., in the hundreds or even higher) yet feel just fine. Other men have low values yet have symptoms of the disease. PSA levels are *not* a definitive measure of how serious one's prostate cancer is and are only part of the information that your doctor uses to determine how you are doing in relation to your prostate cancer.

PSA levels normally fluctuate in all men. Many men dealing with prostate cancer are understandably concerned about even very small changes in their PSA. For men whose cancer has recurred or spread outside the prostate gland, the actual PSA level is typically not as important as how quickly it rises. However, not every rise in PSA means that the cancer is growing and requires treatment right away. To help avoid unnecessary anxiety, be sure you understand what level of change in your PSA is considered a cause for concern. You can determine this by speaking with your doctor.

How Long Will ADT Control My Cancer?

Patients may be treated with ADT for many years, for as long as it is beneficial in managing their cancer. Many men have been on ADT for more than a decade and some have been on and off it for over two decades. ADT works for varying periods of time in different patients. Be sure to discuss with your doctor your questions about the duration of ADT and the potential for intermittent treatment strategies. Intermittent therapy requires regular monitoring of your PSA and overall health to ensure that drug treatment is reinitiated in a timely fashion if necessary. For many patients, intermittent therapy appears to match the benefits of continuous hormonal treatment for prostate cancer control, and is associated with a better quality of life during the "off" treatment periods.

However, over time ADT will likely become less effective at reducing PSA levels. When that happens, other treatments (e.g., second- and third-line therapies) can be considered. Long-term administration of ADT is increasingly offered to patients in the intermittent manner. For some patients the cyclic use of the LHRH drugs may prolong the length of time that the ADT remains effective in controlling the cancer, but data are few to show that intermittent therapy extends life overall.

Hearing that your primary treatment did not get rid of all the cancer or that your cancer has spread can be distressing for both you and your loved ones. At this point, we know that the previous, potentially curative treatment has failed. Some distress is understandable in this situation. These feelings should be balanced against the reality that ADT can help control your cancer for a long time, and patients now on intermittent ADT may go through a half dozen or more "off" cycles, which can sometimes span a decade or longer.

For patients on intermittent ADT, getting PSA tests and waiting for the results are often stressful times. Feeling nervous or anxious is realistic in response to this difficult situation. However, if you find that you are significantly distressed at any time while being treated with ADT—whether on an "on" or "off" cycle—you should consider asking your medical team for help in dealing with the stress. Please share your concerns with your physician or seek professional counseling.

A chart for tracking your PSA scores throughout your treatment is provided in the following text and an additional copy is located in the Appendix on page 159.

PSA Chart: Write down the results from your PSA tests to keep track of any changes.

Date	PSA Level

Date	PSA Level

Date	PSA Level

PSA, prostate-specific antigen.

Moving Forward: Questions for Discussion

- Are there questions that I have about ADT for my healthcare team?
- Am I on continuous or intermittent ADT?
- Do I know my PSA?
- How does getting my PSA checked and waiting for results impact my mood or stress level?

NOTES:

_____

_____

_____

_____

_____

_____

_____

2

PHYSICAL SIDE EFFECTS

Androgen deprivation therapy (ADT) eliminates most of the testosterone in a man's body. This can lead to many physical effects. This chapter covers the various side effects that you may experience and offers suggestions for dealing with them. Some of these effects are similar or even identical to those experienced by women when they reach menopause. Knowing this may help loved ones understand what men on ADT experience.

Hot Flashes

Hot flashes (also called *hot flushes*) are often listed by patients as one of the most bothersome side effects of ADT. In various studies, approximately one quarter of all men on ADT rated hot flashes as the most debilitating side effect that they experienced. As many as 80% of ADT patients experience hot flashes but they have been shown to be more of a problem for younger men and for men who are overweight.

Hot flashes can occur within 3 weeks of starting ADT with a luteinizing hormone-releasing hormone (LHRH) agonist, and typically decrease in frequency over the duration of ADT, just as they commonly decrease over time for women after menopause. The hot flashes come on faster with an LHRH antagonist and are somewhat more frequent and severe with degarelix (an LHRH antagonist) than with leuprolide (an LHRH agonist). However, the degree to which men are bothered by hot flashes is comparable for men treated with either type of ADT, 6 months into treatment. While most men report that they get used to hot flashes and are better able to cope with them over time, some men do not.

Hot flashes feel like waves of heat in the face, head, and upper body. Hot flashes involve the perception of heat and are not actually associated with any substantial increase in body temperature. A hot flash usually lasts for less than 3 minutes, though sometimes it can be longer. You may experience hot flashes multiple times in the day or night. During a hot flash, you may feel uncomfortably warm. A severe hot flash can make you feel very hot and sweaty, and may result in needing a change of clothes or bedding.

Hot flashes are often associated with sweating. When the sweating occurs at night, this is called a *night sweat*. Night sweats can interfere with the *quality* of sleep and lead to daytime fatigue, even if you do not remember your sleep being disrupted by them. Night sweats may not only disrupt your sleep, but may also disrupt the sleep of your partner; that is, if you wake up at night, that may wake up your partner. You may find that you may feel daytime sleepiness. Treatments for hot flashes may help improve sleep quality and reduce daytime fatigue for both of you. Even if you are not sure whether hot flashes are disrupting your sleep, you may want to explore with your physician whether treating hot flashes might help with any fatigue you are experiencing.

A hot flash will pass. When you experience one, it can help to use a cold compress, or fan yourself (paper- and battery-operated handheld fans are easy to use and portable). If hot flashes occur often, wear loose clothing in layers that can be quickly put on or taken off. Hot flashes may also improve if you do the following:

- Quit smoking.
- Reduce the amount of spicy food or hot drinks you consume.
- Keep your room at a cooler temperature and use a fan.
- Use light bedding and/or a towel on your sheets.
- Wear breathable (cotton or merino wool) clothing.
- Take warm, rather than hot, baths and showers.

There is some evidence that acupuncture may help reduce the frequency and duration of hot flashes. However, you may need repeated treatment because the benefit of acupuncture in reducing hot flashes may subside over time.

Eating soy products has been suggested as helping to reduce hot flashes. Other compounds derived from plants (e.g., black cohosh) have also been proposed as "natural" treatments for hot flashes. None, however, have been shown to be effective in properly designed clinical trials. For more information, see Chapter 4 on healthy eating. The research demonstrating effectiveness of these treatments is often drawn from the experiences of women with hot flashes at menopause. Less research has been undertaken with men. Effective treatments for women may or may not be effective for men.

We have heard from some patients that they are actually pleased to experience hot flashes, thinking that it confirms that the ADT is working. However, although it is true that hot flashes are an indication of androgen suppression, it would be a mistake to think that there is a relationship between how many hot flashes one experiences and how effective ADT is in controlling one's cancer. The fact is that there is no direct relationship between hot flash severity or frequency and cancer control with ADT. As such, there is no benefit in enduring hot flashes that disrupt one's quality of life.

If hot flashes or night sweats are distressing to you and/or interfere with your sleep, speak to your doctor about medications that can help. Here are some options to consider (also see the table on p. 20).

Medications

Estradiol, the most common natural estrogen, can be applied in low doses to the skin to stop hot flashes. Medications absorbed through the skin are called **transdermal** and it is through this route that estradiol is most safely absorbed (recall the discussion of blood clot risk associated with oral administration of estrogen in Chapter 1). Many women use transdermal estradiol as part of *hormone replacement therapy* to reduce hot flashes during menopause. It is the decline in estradiol, in both menopause and ADT, that causes hot flashes. Estrogens are commonly thought of as female hormones, but they are present in men too. Men normally have some estradiol in their bodies, which is made directly from their testosterone. The two molecules are quite similar and men generally convert some of their testosterone to estradiol, which normally protects them from hot flashes. Men on ADT have less testosterone to be converted to estradiol; thus, they subsequently get hot flashes. It follows then that the most natural way for a man on ADT to control the hot flashes is to replace the missing estradiol. Several other side effects of ADT are partly or fully due to low estradiol and not necessarily due to low testosterone. Thus, replacing the lost estradiol can reduce some of the other ADT side effects.

Estradiol, however, is available by prescription only and, when taken to deal with the hot flashes, is considered an "off-label" use. That means that the product was never actually licensed for that purpose and, as such, some physicians are justifiably hesitant to prescribe it.

There are two ways to use transdermal estradiol. They are the following:

- Adhesive patches that stick to your skin, applied on your buttocks or belly. The patches last up to a week so you do not need to bother with them for days at a time, but they may irritate the skin or become visible by picking up dye from your clothing. Depending on your body size, age, severity of the hot flashes, and size of patches you are using, you may need more than one patch and may need to change them more often than once a week.
- A gel that you can spread on your arms, legs, or abdomen that is clear and quick-drying, so it is not visible, but must be applied daily. Again, you may find that you need more than a single squirt of the gel to get good control of the hot flashes.

There are some important caveats to using transdermal estradiol to manage hot flashes or, for that matter, other ADT side effects. To start with, this treatment should be used with caution when there is a family history of breast cancer that is hormone-sensitive, as adding back an estrogen is best avoided.

Men should be aware that high-dose estradiol may cause breast or nipple sensitivity. Also, based on what is known about estrogens taken orally at a high dose, we cannot yet definitively rule out the potential risk of blood clots. However, ongoing research in the United Kingdom, which is testing out high-dose transdermal estradiol for ADT (aptly named the PATCH study), has not to date documented any increased incidence of blood clots for patients on transdermal estradiol compared to those on the more common LHRH drugs.

There is also a concern that, with **castration-resistant prostate cancer (CRPC)**, there can be a change in the hormone receptors on the cancer cells. In that situation, estrogens, which may help patients in managing ADT side effects, could start to stimulate cancer cell growth. There is not much research on this, but as a cautionary note, it may be best to stop using transdermal estradiol if there is indication that standard ADT can no longer control the cancer.

On the topic of what is the best dose for using transdermal estradiol to control hot flashes, one should appreciate that the amount of estradiol each patient needs may vary greatly depending on things such as his body size, age, and severity of the hot flashes. Many patients who use transdermal estradiol to control hot flashes struggle unnecessarily to find the "right dose." They should expect this to vary over time and, as good general principle, one should use the least amount of medication that works. We are not aware of any studies that have looked at the upper safety limit for the use of transdermal estradiol in men with prostate cancer. If you plan to use transdermal estradiol, when you get a prostate-specific antigen (PSA) test, you can also request to have your estradiol levels measured. In the absence of any data for men, one can extrapolate from what we know is safe for women. And, if the estradiol level is found to be above what is normal for premenopausal women, it might be wise to reduce the amount you are using.

- **Antidepressants**. Certain antidepressant medications can be used to help control hot flashes. These drugs have the elaborate names of selective serotonin reuptake inhibitors (SSRIs) and serotonin norepinephrine reuptake inhibitors (SNRIs). Despite their primary use as antidepressants, in smaller doses, they have also been found to be helpful in reducing the distress from hot flashes. Taking this kind of medication may have the added bonus of helping with mood, should that also be a concern.

  - Venlafaxine (Effexor®), a commonly prescribed SNRI, has been shown to help with hot flashes, with a response rate of just over 60%, with a dose as low as 25 mg. Other drugs in this class may also be helpful.

- Various SSRIs, such as paroxetine (Paxil®) or fluoxetine (Prozac®), are also occasionally prescribed to help men manage severe hot flashes.
- **Gabapentin** (Neurontin®) is a drug commonly used to treat epilepsy and certain types of chronic pain. It has been shown to be moderately effective in treating hot flashes in men on ADT. However, it has not been shown to be better than the agents mentioned earlier.

There are other drugs as well that have been shown to help reduce hot flashes in women, but have not been well studied in prostate cancer patients on ADT. A couple of these drugs are medroxyprogesterone (Provera®) and megestrol (Megace®). They are derived from another natural female hormone, progesterone. Progesterone-derived medications are best known for being used in birth control pills and to treat certain female cancers.

- **Medroxyprogesterone** is primarily a long-acting birth control agent for women (given as an injected drug known as Depo-Provera®), but has also been used at high doses to lower the libido of sex offenders. The fact that it has to be injected makes it less convenient than a pill or a drug applied to the skin. While progesterone-derived agents can reduce hot flashes, they have other side effects that can add to, rather than reduce, the overall side effects of the LHRH drugs. The optimal dose to use should be the least amount needed to control the hot flashes. There are case reports that **megestrol** has stimulated cancer and, therefore, if it is used to treat hot flashes, the cancer needs to be followed closely for signs of progression. Although it can suppress hot flashes, it also may cause weight gain.

The following table lists prescription drugs used to treat hot flashes.

Some Medications for ADT-Induced Hot Flashes

Generic Name	Trade Name	How Is the Drug Given?	How Often Is the Drug Given?
Estradiol	EstroGel®	Gel	Rubbed on the arm once a day
	Alora®	Patch	Applied weekly or twice weekly on the lower abdomen or buttocks
	Climara®		
	Dermestril®		
	Elleste Solo®		
	Esclim®		
	Menostar®		
	Vivelle-Dot®		
Venlafaxine (SNRI)	Effexor, Pristiq®	Pill	Depends on the dose and formulation

(continued)

Some Medications for ADT-Induced Hot Flashes *(continued)*

Generic Name	Trade Name	How Is the Drug Given?	How Often Is the Drug Given?
Paroxetine (SSRI)	Paxil, Pexeva®	Pill	Depends on the dose and formulation
Fluoxetine (SSRI)	Prozac, Sarafem®, Selfemra®	Pill	Depends on the dose and formulation
Gabapentin	Neurontin	Pill	Depends on the dose and formulation
Medroxyprogesterone	Provera	Intramuscular injection into the thigh, abdomen, or arm	One injection every 3 mo
Megestrol	Megace	Pill	Depends on the dose and formulation

SNRI, serotonin norepinephrine reuptake inhibitor; SSRI, selective serotonin reuptake inhibitor.
Note: A low-dose form of paroxetine (Brisdelle) is the only nonhormone treatment for hot flashes approved by the Food and Drug Administration. Other antidepressants that have been used to treat hot flashes include SNRI (Venlafaxine [Effexor XR, Pristiq]) and the SSRIs (Paroxetine [Paxil, Pexeva] and Fluoxetine [Prozac, Sarafem, Selfemra, others]).

Counseling

Counseling approaches such as *cognitive behavioral therapy* can also help you better adjust to the distress (e.g., panic or anger) of experiencing a hot flash and to deal with any negative opinions you might have about what it means as a male to experience a hot flash. The abdominal breathing exercise that follows is one example of a behavioral technique that has been shown to help cope with hot flashes. The hot flash diary on page 22 is an example of a cognitive technique for coping with distressing thoughts about hot flashes. It may at first seem counter-intuitive that documenting bothersome hot flashes by keeping a log can actually reduce the distress associated with the hot flashes. The mechanism behind this is not the recording itself, but rather working to shift or adapt the beliefs you have associated with the experience of a hot flash. Negative beliefs about hot flashes only serve to increase the distress associated with them. There is some data to support this—at least for postmenopausal women.

Activity: Abdominal Breathing

One technique used to reduce hot flash distress is called *abdominal breathing,* or *paced respiration,* which can be used both to reduce the frequency of hot flashes and as a relaxation technique. This type of breathing is most effective after you have practiced it regularly:

- Sit comfortably and place one hand on your belly and one on your chest.
- When you are breathing deeply and slowly, you will find that your belly moves up and down more than if you were taking shallow breaths.
- When you are ready, take a deep breath in through your nose. Make this inhalation last for a count of four, and then pause. Breathe out through your nose, exhaling out all the breath while slowly counting to four, and then pause. Inhale. Exhale. Inhale. Exhale. Try doing this for a few minutes.
- Be sure to focus on your breath. If you notice thoughts coming and going, acknowledge them and try to bring your attention back to your breath. Try not to allow yourself to be frustrated when your mind wanders. If you get overwhelmed, tired, or dizzy at first, take a break for about 30 seconds and continue when you are ready. It helps to concentrate on slowly filling and emptying your lungs as fully as is possible.

With continued practice (daily, for 5 minutes at a time), you can get better at this activity. It can be an effective and simple way to cope with a hot flash when one comes on assuming you have previously practiced the exercise. This is also an effective strategy for coping with anxiety and stress, discussed further in Chapter 5.

Activity: Hot Flash Diary

You may find a hot flash diary to be helpful for tracking the frequency of your hot flashes, how bothersome they are to you, and how you will cope with them. Sometimes the thoughts that come with hot flashes can be as distressing as the hot flash itself. For example, if you think, "Oh no, I can't cope with this hot flash," this mere thought can perpetuate distress. It may be helpful to challenge this thought or remind yourself of a coping statement. Examples of these include the following:

"There are things I can do to cope with this discomfort, such as deep breathing."
"The people I am with right now know what I am going through and are not going to make fun of me for having a hot flash."
"I can ask my doctor about medications to help with hot flashes."
"Yes a hot flash is uncomfortable, but I can handle it, it will be over soon."

Coping statements give a rational perspective on the situation and are helpful in handling momentary distress. They help keep distressing thoughts in check and prevent a person from becoming overwhelmed by them. Keeping a record of your hot flashes can help increase objectivity and thus decrease distress. The hot flash diary follows, and can also be found in the Appendix on page 160.

Hot Flash Diary

Day	Intensity (0–10)	Duration	Distressing Thought/ Appraisal	Coping Statement
Sunday				
Monday				
Tuesday				
Wednesday				
Thursday				
Friday				
Saturday				

Weaker Bones

ADT can affect how strong your bones are. Slight weakening of bones is called *osteopenia*; more extensive weakening is called **osteoporosis**. With weaker bones, the risk of breaking a bone is increased with relatively minor trauma, including falls.

If there is a history of osteoporosis or hip fractures for your parents, you may be at especially high risk of a fracture while on ADT. ADT has independently been linked to not only a heightened risk of osteoporosis but an actual increase in falling, and fracturing a bone if you fall. Thus, the risk from osteoporosis is not just hypothetical; it is something that men on ADT must be attentive to. The risk of osteoporosis increases the longer one is on ADT, so before or soon after starting ADT discuss with your doctor what actions you can take to reduce your risk of osteoporosis.

Here are some things to consider to prevent osteoporosis and the risk of a bone fracture if you are starting on ADT:

- Individuals may not know that they have osteoporosis until they actually break a bone. However, one can get a baseline bone density exam to measure **bone mineral density (BMD)**. BMD measurement is how osteopenia and osteoporosis are formally assessed. The higher your BMD, the stronger your bones are.

  BMD is measured with an x-ray called **dual-energy x-ray absorptiometry**. This is usually just abbreviated to **DEXA**. With DEXA, double x-ray images are taken. This allows the machine to subtract the image of soft tissue from the image of the bones. The BMD can then be determined from the x-ray data on the bones themselves.
  - A DEXA scan is simple, noninvasive, and can be repeated over time to assess the impact of ADT on your bone health. It should be noted that most bone density exams are not sensitive enough to pick up changes in men on ADT for a short term, such as 6 months or less. You thus need to discuss with your physician if the scan is worth getting given your personal history, family history, and the length of time you are likely to be on ADT. If you are going to be on ADT long term, it may be a good idea to get a DEXA scan every year or two.
- See Chapter 3 on exercise for activities that will help strengthen bones and improve muscle strength and balance. There are solid data to show that resistance training and specifically impact loading can improve BMD for men on ADT.
- Stop smoking and limit alcohol and caffeine consumption.
- Strive to maintain a healthy weight.
- Talk to your doctor about taking calcium and vitamin D supplementation. You should aim for 1500 to 2000 **IU** (International Units) of vitamin D a day (described in more detail in Chapter 4).
- Bisphosphonates are a class of drugs commonly used to treat osteoporosis and may be used to counteract the effects of ADT on your bones. These agents may also be helpful in managing prostate cancer that has spread to your bones. Bisphosphonate drugs can be administered orally (e.g., alendronate, brand name Fosamax®) and intravenously (e.g., zoledronic acid, brand name Zometa®) but the intravenous ones are stronger drugs. Like any medication, there are potential side effects and risks associated with the use of bisphosphonates that you should be aware of and discuss with your doctor before starting on such drugs. These medications are not often used preemptively for all patients starting on ADT, but rather may be introduced when bone density exams reveal a drop in bone density, or may be used more commonly with men who are going to be on long-term ADT.
- If you are starting on drugs to protect your bones while on ADT, it is important to make your dentist aware and to have a dental assessment because of a rare, yet potentially serious and painful side effect called *osteonecrosis of the jaw* (ONJ). ONJ is death of the bone in your jaw following some infection. The infection usually begins with major dental work. Your dentist can take

precautions to reduce the risk of ONJ and it is suggested that you have your dental work up to date before you start on bisphosphonate medication.

- Long-term use (e.g., ≥5 years) of bisphosphonates for postmenopausal women has been shown to occasionally lead to a rare form of fracture of the hip or thigh. If you are taking a bisphosphonate for a long time and experience hip or thigh pain, be sure to bring that to the attention of your physician.
- Using transdermal estradiol to reduce hot flashes may also help keep your bones strong. The evidence for this comes from the clinical trial in the United Kingdom using high-dose transdermal estradiol for ADT. It is also consistent with data from women who are at risk of developing osteoporosis when their estrogen levels decline at menopause.
- Denosumab (Xgeva®) is a different class of drug than the bisphosphonates, but is similarly used to help manage bone health in patients at risk of osteoporosis and cancer that is affecting their bones. Denosumab is given as an injection once every 6 months for men with osteoporosis. However, for patients whose cancer has spread (i.e., is metastatic) it may be given more often, such as once a month, for as long as it is needed. It can, however, interfere with immune function, slightly increasing the risk of respiratory or bladder infections and, like the bisphosphonates, it carries a similar risk of ONJ.

Weight Gain and Muscle Loss

Weight gain is a common complaint of many men who are treated with ADT. The gain is largely due to an increase in the amount of fat men store in the body while on these drugs. This weight gain occurs in about 70% of men on ADT. Most of the fat is added to the belly and some to the hips. You are most likely to experience this increase in weight in the first year of ADT, particularly if you are not very physically active.

Different studies give various numbers for the average amount gained as fat, but 5 to 10 pounds (up to 4.2 kg) is not uncommon. Younger men, and men who are of normal weight or slightly overweight but not obese, are at greatest risk of gaining weight as fat. At the same time, there are some men who actually lose weight while on ADT.

If you are presently at a normal or low weight, weight gain of this amount may not be serious. However, if you are already overweight, relatively inactive, or at risk of developing diabetes, then weight gain may be problematic.

Well-structured exercise programs are prescribed treatments for many medical conditions. Unless you have been told by your doctor not to exercise, we encourage you to view an exercise program as a significant part of your treatment regimen while on ADT. We recognize that starting a program now may not be easy, but its benefits are many!

Physical Side Effects

Increases in weight while on ADT can lead to medical complications, such as diabetes and cardiac problems (called **metabolic syndrome**).

Although ADT is typically associated with a weight gain as fat, there is commonly a cooccurring loss of 3% to 4% of muscle mass. The combination of muscle loss (called **sarcopenia**) and an increase in weight as fat (together called sarcopenic obesity) makes moving more difficult . . . and being inactive just makes matters worse. If you are not already exercising consistently, try increasing your activity level gradually. If you find yourself gaining a lot of weight, one of the best things you can do is maintain a regular exercise schedule. Even if you do not lose the fat, the exercise will help preserve muscle strength and balance, reducing your risk of a fall. See Chapter 3 on exercise for more information. Suggestions for implementing your exercise routine include the following:

- Joining a structured program at a gym or community center.
- Purchasing equipment to use at home, such as small free weights and stretchable bands.

> **It is important that you do not wait until you notice changes in weight and muscle mass before you begin an exercise program. Once you gain weight, it can be more difficult to lose it. So start now! You may find it more enjoyable to pursue an exercise program with your partner, a friend, or a loved one.**

Diabetes

ADT not only increases the risk of adult onset (type 2) diabetes, but has also recently been found to make the control of diabetes with medications alone more difficult. Thus, prostate cancer patients who are diabetic and starting on ADT need to be particularly concerned about their lifestyle—that is, diet and exercise—if they are going to keep their diabetes under control and avoid the more serious complications of that disease.

Active research is underway to find out whether patients on ADT do better if given metformin, a common drug used to treat diabetes. Although not all the results are in yet, a patient on ADT, who is already diabetic or at particularly high risk of developing that disease, may want to discuss with his physician the pros and cons of taking metformin while on ADT. *However*, taking such a drug is *not* a replacement for exercising. As noted earlier, the effectiveness of such drugs is already known to be better for patients who are actively exercising.

Metabolic Syndrome and Cardiovascular Risk

ADT has been shown to cause metabolic abnormalities. Metabolic syndrome is diagnosed when there are at least three of the following five symptoms: increased blood sugar (6.105 mmol/L or >110 mg/dL), increased triglycerides (1.695 mmol/L or ≥150 mg/dL or higher), low high-density lipoproteins (1.036 mmol/L or <40 mg/dL), increased waist circumference of 40 inches (102 cm), and/or increased blood pressure (≥130/85 mmHg or higher). The blood sugar triglycerides and lipoprotein profiles are assessed from blood drawn during a standard blood test.

Men on ADT often experience an increase in blood sugar, triglycerides, and waist circumference. Collectively, these are markers of increased risk of developing both diabetes and cardiovascular disease. Metabolic syndrome is an example of the more serious side effects that can come with ADT, yet are not obvious to patients without blood tests and a clinical checkup. The risk of metabolic syndrome can emerge within a year or two of starting on ADT for patients who have not taken precautions to limit it.

With exercise and diet, the shift in the blood profile and waist circumference toward metabolic syndrome can be slowed down or even stopped. Chapters 3 and 4 cover the type of exercise and diet that can protect you from metabolic syndrome and the more serious diseases that can follow that.

As already mentioned earlier, there is active research underway on adding metformin, a drug to treat diabetes, to ADT for men at risk of metabolic syndrome and subsequent diabetes. In a similar vein, there is research underway exploring the preemptive use of medications to reduce the risk of cardiovascular disease for men on ADT. Two of the drugs under study are low-dose aspirin and drugs called statins, which are cholesterol-lowering agents. The statins include atorvastatin, fluvastatin, lovastatin, pitavastatin, pravastatin, rosuvastatin, and simvastatin. The most common brand names are Lipitor® (atorvastatin) and Crestor® (rosuvastatin), but they are available now as generic drugs and the generics are typically cheaper than the brand name products.

All of these drugs have their own side effects, which you need to be aware of if you are starting on any of them. Increasingly physicians who start patients on ADT assess patients' cardiovascular health, to look for preexisting conditions such as metabolic syndrome, diabetes, and previous cardiovascular events. They use that to help decide whether you are likely to benefit from additional medications.

Cardiovascular disease is not one disease and the risks of getting any one of the many diseases that fit in that category vary greatly. Racial background may also affect cardiovascular risk with ADT; thus, those of an Asian, African, or European background can expect different risks. All of this needs to be taken into consideration if one is going to take additional medications when on ADT.

Of the various cardiovascular diseases, blockage of the vessels that provide blood to the heart itself are the ones of most concern. Such blockage is typically caused by atherosclerotic plaque formation, which is a buildup of fatty material in the walls of those vessels and thus narrows the vessels, limiting blood flow through them. In serious cases, they can lead to a complete blockage of the vessels that in turn deprives the heart muscle of oxygen. That can lead to heart pain (angina) and, in the worst situation, the heart muscle normally supplied by the blocked vessel can die (formally called an *acute myocardial infarction*, but most people know it as a heart attack). If the plaque breaks off and moves through the vessels to the brain, that is what is known as a stroke. Both are very serious.

The risk of either condition arising with ADT appears to be related to the amount of plaque in the vessels before one starts on ADT. One study suggests that men who have had a heart attack in the year before starting on ADT are at further increased risk of a heart attack or stroke in the first year of being on ADT, at least with the standard LHRH agonists. There is some evidence, though, that the risk might be slightly lower with degarelix, an LHRH antagonist, or possibly with an orchiectomy.

One should be aware of the characteristics of a heart attack. This can be felt as a deep crushing pain in the chest, but this pain can also radiate to the left shoulder and upper part of the left arm. If you have experienced anything like that, you should tell your doctor about it whether you are on ADT or not.

Anemia and Fatigue

From a third to a half of men on ADT experience some level of daytime fatigue, that is, the feeling of lacking energy and motivation mentally and/or physically. This effect seems to be felt more by younger men, since they experience a greater drop in testosterone. There are several factors that can lead to the sense of fatigue. Some of them have already been mentioned, such as disrupted sleep from hot flashes, and a feeling that normal activities take more effort secondary to sarcopenia.

You may be suffering from night sweats (hot flashes) that are disrupting your sleep. There is also mental fatigue associated with ADT (see Chapter 5). As a result, you may feel less motivated to exercise or participate in physical activities. You may also get out of breath more quickly when you are physically active. You may not feel like exercising because you are too tired, *but the single best way to combat fatigue from ADT is through exercise*.

If you are taking abiraterone or enzalutamide, your fatigue could be more severe than that of patients who are receiving other ADT drugs. This is because abiraterone is more effective in lowering the androgen in the body than other ADT drugs, and enzalutamide can effectively block androgens from having any effects on cells. Starting exercise can be even more challenging while on these drugs, but you may try by starting a small amount of exercise first, and gradually increase the frequency and duration over time.

Avoiding exercise is a vicious circle: You will lose muscle mass and gain weight, which makes you feel more tired and even less enthusiastic about exercising. You may feel that exercising is not helping; you may still gain weight and lose muscle mass despite exercising. That does not mean that exercise is not preventing things from being much worse. Read Chapter 3 on exercise and talk with your physician to find an exercise program that is best for you.

ADT can cause mild anemia, which means there are fewer than normal red blood cells and an abnormally low amount of the molecule hemoglobin in those cells. Hemoglobin transports oxygen from the lungs to the rest of the body. That oxygen is necessary for numerous body functions and with low hemoglobin many activities take more effort. This is experienced as fatigue. Women usually have slightly less hemoglobin than men. Hemoglobin is commonly measured in grams per deciliter (= g/dL), with the normal range for men being 13.5 to 17.5 and 12.0 to 15.5 for women. (This is sometimes presented in **SI** units called millimoles per litre [= mmol/L] where the normal range for men is 8.38 to 10.86 and 7.45 to 9.62 for women.). The hemoglobin of men on ADT may shift to the range known for women, but rarely is that large enough to be a major source of fatigue.

ADT-associated anemia is *not* due to an iron deficiency and taking an iron supplement is *not* recommended unless you are iron deficient. However, if you are experiencing extreme fatigue while on ADT, you should inform your doctor. Although ADT does not itself lead to iron deficiency anemia, one can have anemia from iron deficiency or other reasons independent of any mild anemia due to ADT.

Regular exercise reduces fatigue, keeps muscles strong, and limits weight gain. It promotes an all-around better mood during the day and helps improve sleep quality.

Breast Growth

Approximately 15% of patients taking LHRH agonists experience some level of breast enlargement and increased breast or nipple sensitivity. Such breast growth in men is called **gynecomastia**. The amount of breast growth is usually slight, but the nipples and surrounding skin may become more sensitive to touch. Pain and discomfort in the nipples or breast is called **mastalgia**. Gynecomastia is more common in patients taking antiandrogen medications that may be prescribed to enhance ADT effectiveness. Breast development is also common in patients who use low-dose estradiol to reduce hot flashes or high-dose transdermal estradiol for androgen suppression. Some patients find that they are uncomfortable with the changes in appearance or nipple sensitivity that accompany gynecomastia. There is no definitive way to predict who will experience these symptoms, but if you are overweight, your chances may be greater.

Men vary greatly in how bothered they are by gynecomastia. For most men, breasts are a signifier of feminization, so any enlargement of their breasts might be seen as loss of masculinity, identity, and status. For some men gynecomastia is shameful and distressing. Other men are not bothered by the changes.

Some men even find the fact that they have gynecomastia amusing. If you stop ADT, breast sensitivity may stop, but the breast tissue itself will not disappear.

If you are distressed by gynecomastia, you can do the following:

- Wear a T-shirt at the gym or beach, or a wetsuit vest in the water.
- Exercise at home by investing in personal fitness equipment.
- Invest in garments that compress and flatten the chest, such as compression shirts—some common brands include Nike®, Under Armour®, and InstaSlim®.

One man on ADT was able to joke about his breast development, teasing his wife that his breasts were younger and better looking than hers.

It is important that you and your intimate partner discuss what gynecomastia would mean to each of you. If you think that breast development will be very distressing to you, or that you cannot tolerate it at all, discuss preventative options with your doctor as soon as possible. Unfortunately, such procedures may not be covered by your health insurance.

There is a drug used to treat breast cancer, called tamoxifen, which is technically a selective estrogen-receptor modulator (SERM) and sold as a generic product or under the brand names of Nolvadex®, Istubal®, or Valodex®. Tamoxifen has been suggested as a drug to limit the risk of gynecomastia for men on ADT treatments that are most likely to cause breast growth such as antiandrogen or estradiol monotherapy. However, there have not been long-term studies on the benefits or risks of taking an SERM to block estrogenic effects associated with various forms of ADT.

You should thus consult with your physician before taking tamoxifen because SERMs can influence the various effects of estrogen in the body, and tamoxifen has its own side effects. Some research suggests though that most men, who are exceptionally bothered by gynecomastia, can tolerate the side effects of tamoxifen.

Some of the more established options to prevent or reduce gynecomastia include the following:

- Preemptive *irradiation of the breasts:* In order to be most effective, this treatment should be undertaken *before* gynecomastia develops. The radiation decreases potential breast growth, and, to some extent, may help to reduce breast sensitivity and discomfort.
- *Breast reduction surgery:* If breast growth is very distressing, breast reduction surgery is an option, and in some cases may be covered by health insurance. There are various ways that this surgery can be performed.

When it is performed for men for strictly cosmetic reasons, it can usually be done as a nipple-sparing (subcutaneous) mastectomy or with liposuction.

Genital Shrinkage

With ADT, some shrinkage of the penis and testicles is common. The shrinkage of the testicles is directly related to the shutdown of their functions of producing testosterone and sperm. If you are on ADT short term (<3 years), the size of your testicles can mostly recover when your testosterone levels recover. Since the testicles are inside the scrotum and not externally visible, their shrinkage is usually less of an issue for men on ADT compared to the loss of penis length and girth.

If you have residual **erectile dysfunction (ED)** from an earlier treatment for prostate cancer (e.g., surgery or radiation), you may have already experienced some shrinkage of your penis. The loss on average is about 2 centimeters in the first year and about 0.7 centimeters in the second year, but stabilizes after that.

Along with a decrease in sex drive, men on ADT often lose the ability to have a strong and prolonged erection, including spontaneous erections such as nocturnal erections. Just as the muscles in an arm will shrink if the arm is not actively moved, the penis will shrink if erections become rare or disappear completely. Most often these changes occur slowly and may not be noticeable for many months.

> **Whether or not you and your partner intend to engage in penile penetrative sex, it is worth considering the impact that genital shrinkage will have on your self-image. Men vary greatly in how much their penis size means to their self-image.**

Penile shrinkage combined with increased abdominal fat may make it more difficult to see the penis and accurately aim while urinating. If that becomes a problem, the solution is to urinate sitting down.

Genital shrinkage does not often get discussed with patients, but it is common among men who are on ADT long term. Men's responses to genital shrinkage vary greatly. To some it is of no concern, while for others it is a major concern. Sexual partners respond differently as well. Even though many partners indicate that penis size does not matter to them, they should appreciate that it can be an emotionally charged issue for some men.

If you do not envision participating in the future in sexual activities that depend on penile erections, penis size and function may not be an issue for you. Still, you may be concerned about how your penis looks or feels to you, even if function is not an issue. For some men, such an alteration can really affect their self-esteem. If distress about this change prevents you from living well and especially from going to the gym or the swimming pool, schedule your exercise program so you can shower and dress in private.

If penis size is important to you, and if your hormone treatment is short term, and if you envision resuming intercourse when you are off of ADT, you may want to read about options to maintain penis size and/or function in the absence of erections. Several management strategies are available, including ways to create erections regularly (such as the use of a vacuum erection device [VED] or penile injection) that can help keep the penile tissues from shrinking. There is some suggestion that, for men on short-term ADT, regular use of the VED while on ADT can help reduce the shrinkage. For information on the VED see Chapter 6. Certain ED treatments, specifically penile implant and those that involve injecting drugs directly into the penis, can produce erections even in the absence of strong sexual desire. It should be acknowledged, though, that in the absence of a strong libido, such artificially induced erections may feel mechanical and unnatural to a patient.

You and your sexual partner may wish to research ED treatments. We encourage you to read the whole chapter on intimacy and sexuality, starting on page 105. It is important to note that not all men who try these strategies find them helpful or effective.

Loss of Body Hair

Men on ADT typically lose the hair on their chest, back, arms, and legs. Hair in the armpits and facial hair may be reduced in density, but hair on the top of the head and pubic hair remain. There are no physical health implications to losing body hair, and there is no easy way to stop it. Be aware that many men nowadays spend a lot of effort shaving and waxing to remove body hair, and men vary enormously on how hairy their bodies are to begin with. Thus, reduced body hair may even go unnoticed by those other than yourself or intimate partners.

Other Possible Side Effects

The official pharmaceutical literature on the LHRH agonists and antagonists lists a large array of other physical side effects that have been infrequently reported by patients on ADT. These occur in fewer than 10% of patients. Many of them are required to be listed by the national agencies that authorize the licensing of the drugs in different countries even though a causal link to ADT has not been established.

Such symptoms are ones that we all may experience at various times in our lives and are common illnesses. Here are a few examples that fit that pattern: headache, upset stomach, nausea, diarrhea, constipation, and joint/muscle aches or pains. Many of these occur at about the same frequency for people who are not on ADT. Others are so rare that they were only identified from studies with very large sample sizes. A few of these, though rare, are also serious, and are thus worth some attention.

One recent study suggests that patients on ADT have a slightly increased risk of acute kidney failure. That risk may be a bit higher for those on LHRH agonists than patients who are surgically castrated. There are standard blood tests that physicians use to tell how healthy your kidneys are and the risk of kidney failure. With acute kidney failure, the kidneys stop working and, along with other symptoms, there can be dangerous levels of fluid retention in the body. As such, you may want to request that indicators of kidney function be included when you get your regular PSA blood tests.

Another potentially serious side effect, but also considered very rare, is an increased risk of colorectal cancer with long-term use of ADT. The United States and Canada, as well as most other industrial countries, have national guidelines on how often one should be screened for colorectal cancer once they have passed the age of 50. We encourage men on ADT to review those guidelines with their physician and get screened at the frequency recommended—following, of course, their physician's advice.

Another recent study found that ADT is associated with a slight increased risk of developing a lung infection, that is, pneumonia. While ADT may not directly cause pneumonia, the researchers who discovered this link suggested that the loss of androgen may impair the immune system, making patients on ADT more prone to lung infection. This is consistent with the fact that autoimmune diseases are more common in women than men, although there is not much evidence that ADT impairs the immune system in general. More research is needed to confirm that any link between ADT and pneumonia is due to changes in the immune system. Furthermore, although asthma has not been linked to ADT, there are some data to suggest that testosterone helps protect men from that respiratory condition.

There are other equally credible hypotheses that could account for an association of ADT with the risk of pneumonia. For example, one of the natural mechanisms that protects us from lung infections is to have a strong cough that can clear our lungs of bacteria and viruses. Coughing requires contracting the muscles of the body wall. Since ADT can lead to loss of muscle strength, it is possible that patients on ADT who experience muscle loss in the core, chest, or abdomen may be at heightened risk of that respiratory problem.

Another condition that seems to appear more often in men on ADT is periodontal disease. As a precaution, patients on ADT should take good care of their teeth and gums.

On an interesting note, one side effect that scientists are just now investigating is a subtle change in body odor. This is simply mentioned here for thoroughness.

Perhaps the most common, but rather nonspecific, effect that patients report while on ADT is some joint or muscle pain. As men get older general aches and pains in muscles and joints are increasingly common. They may be due to factors such as arthritis and stiffness secondary to inactivity. There is not a lot of evidence to support the view that they are directly caused by ADT. As noted in Chapter 5, ADT is associated with increased risk of anxiety and/or depression. It is possible that the experience of aches and pains can be influenced by anxiety or depression, such as being overly attentive to otherwise minor aches and pains, making them seem progressively worse. Our mood and how our body feels may influence each other at any time. The topic of ADT's effect on mood is taken up in much greater detail in Chapter 5.

If muscle or joint discomfort persists and gets worse while you are on ADT, these issues should be brought to the attention of your doctor. They may be unrelated to prostate cancer or its treatment and may reflect some new health issue that needs to be properly assessed. For example, they may be the result of the side effects of other medications or supplements that you are taking. So when you talk to your healthcare providers about any medical issues, be sure to bring with you a list of the medications and supplements you are taking.

Collectively, the chances of serious diseases, such as kidney failure or pneumonia, are extremely rare. Unfortunately, such diseases, along with general aches and pains, come with aging regardless of whether one is on ADT or not. Once again, assuming that these conditions are not related to some other causes, the best intervention for dealing with them is to stay physically active.

Activity: Pros/Cons Table

Managing the side effects of androgen deprivation therapy (ADT) often requires making substantial changes to one's lifestyle. Sometimes, even though you *want* to make a lifestyle change, you may need to persuade yourself that the change is in fact worthwhile. A Pros/Cons table is a great way to convince yourself of the importance of making a change. You can redo it anytime you feel as if your life and priorities have shifted. Here is an example of a table:

	PROS	CONS
MAKING THE CHANGE: Walking daily	• Becoming fit • Feeling better about myself • Being outdoors • Treats fatigue • Helps treat muscle mass loss	• Requires effort • Takes up time • Tiring
STAYING THE SAME: Stay at the same level of physical activity	• Easier to just enjoy myself and relax/sit on my couch • Not tiring • More time for other things	• I will probably gain weight • I am just so tired

Now, try it out for yourself. An additional copy is in the Appendix on page 161.

	PROS	CONS

MAKING THE CHANGE:

STAYING THE SAME:

Activity: Action Plan

Throughout this book, there are suggestions for change that will help you and your partner maintain a high quality of life while on ADT. Are you thinking about making a lifestyle change? Eating better? Exercising more? Spending more time communicating with your partner? An *Action Plan* is a structured way to help you be clear about your goals, and increase the likelihood that you will follow through on your plans. It helps to be specific about when and where you plan to do the particular activity. You may wish to start small with something very manageable (e.g., going to the gym twice a week) before you take on larger scale goals (e.g., going to the gym every day). Discussing your Action Plan with a close friend or family member may help to keep you on track with your goals. Here is an example of a completed Action Plan:

Action Plan Example: Practice Abdominal Breathing to Help With Hot Flashes

What I plan to do: try abdominal breathing for hot flashes

When I plan to do it: twice a day before lunch and dinner

Who I might do it with: by myself

Where I plan to do it: at my desk before lunch and/or in my living room before dinner

Why my plan is important: to help myself cope with discomfort

What might get in the way? forgetting

How I will address what might get in the way: I will put it in my daytimer, or set a smartphone reminder

Here is a blank copy that you can fill out. It helps to be as specific as possible when you are making your Action Plan. An additional copy is available in the Appendix on page 162.

Action Plan: _____

What I plan to do: _____
_____

When I plan to do it: _____
_____

Who I might do it with: _____
_____

Where I plan to do it: _____
_____

Why my plan is important: _____
_____

What might get in the way: _____
_____

How I will address what might get in the way: _____
_____

Activity: Goal Setting and Confidence

In order to support your goal, it can be helpful to ask yourself how confident you are that you can be successful in making this change. First, write down your goal (this might be what you have written in your Action Plan):

GOAL #1 _____

  i) Rate how confident you feel that you will achieve your goal:
     1   2   3   4   5   6   7   8   9   10
     Not confident   Very confident
  ii) Rate how motivated you are to accomplish your goal:
     1   2   3   4   5   6   7   8   9   10
     Not motivated   Very motivated
  iii) Rate how likely you are to actually carry out your goal:
     1   2   3   4   5   6   7   8   9   10
     Not likely   Very likely

If any of your answers *are less than five*:

- Some ways to enhance motivation: (a) Consider enlisting the help of a friend to hold you accountable, (b) set up a reward system, so that when you have achieved the goal, you can reward yourself, (c) review a list of the possible benefits that may come from this change in behavior.
- Consider revising your goal—is it too ambitious? Can you start with a more modest goal and work your way up to a more significant lifestyle change?
- Remind yourself—What are the reasons why you are motivated to make this change?
- Consider completing the previous Pros/Cons table to help you identify your motivations (pros) for making this change, but also some of the barriers (cons) that might be getting in the way of making the change.

Activity: Side Effects Self-Assessment

It is hard to adapt to changes one does not see or recognize. Thus, it is important to keep track of your side effects. Most of the side effects listed in the text that follows were discussed in this chapter, though a few are detailed more in Chapters 5 to 7. Awareness of change is always an aid in adapting to change. Use the following questionnaire to help you recognize the impact of ADT on your life. Many of these side effects will take some time to develop; therefore, you may find it helpful to complete this brief assessment *after* you have been on ADT for 3 months. Fill it out and show it to your healthcare provider at your next appointment so that any concerns you have can be addressed. You may find it helpful to fill out the questionnaire before each of your medical appointments.

For descriptions and management strategies of the side effects listed in the following text, see the appropriate chapter. You can find an additional copy of the side effects assessment in the Appendix on pages 164 to 165.

1. **During the past month**, how often have you experienced hot flashes? (*Please circle one number.*)
   - (1) More than once a day
   - (2) About once a day
   - (3) More than once a week
   - (4) About once a week
   - (5) Rarely or never

2. **During the past month**, how often have you had breast tenderness/sensitivity? (*Please circle one number.*)
   - (1) More than once a day
   - (2) About once a day
   - (3) More than once a week
   - (4) About once a week
   - (5) Rarely or never

3. **During the past month**, have you noticed any breast enlargement? (*Please circle one number.*)
   (1) None
   (2) Minimal
   (3) Substantial
   (4) Moderate

4. **During the past month**, how much has your weight changed, if at all? (*Please circle one number.*)
   (1) Gained 5 lb./2.3 kg or more
   (2) Gained less than 5 lb./2.3 kg
   (3) No change in weight
   (4) Lost less than 5 lb./2.3 kg
   (5) Lost 5 lb./2.3 kg or more

5. **During the past month**, have you noticed a change in the amount of hair on your arms, legs, and torso? (*Please circle one number.*)
   (1) Loss of body hair on arms, legs, and/or torso
   (2) No loss of body hair

6. **During the past month**, how concerned have you been about changes in how your penis and scrotum look? (*Please circle one number.*)
   (1) Not concerned at all
   (2) A little concerned
   (3) Moderately concerned
   (4) Highly concerned

7. **During the past month**, how has your level of sexual desire been? (*Please circle one number.*)
   (1) Very low to none
   (2) Low
   (3) Moderate
   (4) High
   (5) Very high

8. **During the past month**, how has your ability to have an erection been? (*Please circle one number.*)
   (1) Very poor to none
   (2) Poor
   (3) Fair
   (4) Good
   (5) Very good/excellent

9. **During the past month**, how often have you experienced a problem remembering something that you thought you knew well? (*Please circle one number.*)
   (1) More than once a day
   (2) About once a day
   (3) More than once a week
   (4) About once a week
   (5) Rarely or never

10. **During the past month**, how often have you felt sad or depressed? (*Please circle one number.*)
    (1) More than once a day
    (2) About once a day
    (3) More than once a week
    (4) About once a week
    (5) Rarely or never

11. **During the past month**, how often have you felt a lack of energy? (*Please circle one number.*)
    (1) More than once a day
    (2) About once a day
    (3) More than once a week
    (4) About once a week
    (5) Rarely or never

Physical Side Effects: Essentials

The physical side effects of ADT can be divided into two major categories: (a) those that affect how your body feels (e.g., hot flashes, loss of muscle strength, fatigue) and (b) those that affect how your body appears (e.g., loss of body hair, gynecomastia, genital shrinkage). Weight gain affects both how your body looks and feels. All of these changes may affect the patient and indirectly his loved ones emotionally. Most patients are likely to experience some, but not necessarily all, side effects.

From a medical perspective, the side effects of greatest concern are those that affect your overall physical health, such as weight gain, bone loss, and metabolic syndrome. Being inactive and overweight increases the risk of other serious illnesses, such as diabetes and cardiovascular disease (leading to heart attack or stroke). Bone loss in turn increases the risk of fracture. You should be aware of these concerns and engage in activities and treatments that can help limit the negative impact of ADT on your overall health.

Exercise and a proper diet are ways to deal with potentially serious complications of ADT. Together they are proven to maintain good health and overall quality of life for patients on ADT. We strongly urge you to incorporate an exercise program into your normal weekly routines *before* you experience the full impact of ADT.

The side effects of ADT can interact with one another. For example, hot flashes that disrupt your sleep can make you tired and less motivated to exercise. But by not exercising, you can gain weight, lose bone density, and increase your risk of other serious illnesses.

The side effects that alter male appearance (e.g., gynecomastia, loss of body hair) tend to feminize the body. Patients on ADT do not lose facial hair nor does the pitch of the voice change noticeably; thus, these physical changes do not substantially alter key markers of the male sex. However, you may be bothered by such changes. If you are having difficulty coping with changes in your appearance, consider seeking the help of a professional counselor. Another key to success is to keep communication open with your partner, supportive family members and friends, and, most importantly, with your doctor. Open communication helps to facilitate adapting to any ADT-related changes.

Moving Forward: Questions for Discussion

Here are a few questions to help you think about what you learned in this chapter and how it may affect you. Encourage your partner or loved ones to answer these questions too, and discuss your answers with one another. Writing out your answers, and any other questions that may arise from thinking about these topics, is also recommended.

- Of all the physical side effects, the ones I am most concerned about are . . .
- The side effects that I think my partner might be most concerned about are . . .
- What are some of the potential solutions I might be willing to try in order to reduce the impact of that side effect?
- Could it help to talk to members of a support group about ADT or to another patient who has experienced ADT firsthand?
- Am I getting enough physical activity? How can I incorporate exercise (cardio, strength training, and flexibility) into my daily life?
- What things can I ask my partner or friends to help me with, in adjusting to the physical side effects of ADT?

NOTES:

_____
_____
_____
_____
_____
_____
_____
_____
_____
_____

3

EXERCISE

Current guidelines for all cancer survivors recommend 150 minutes of moderate to vigorously intense exercise per week. Because of androgen deprivation therapy (ADT) side effects, it is especially important for men on ADT to strive for regular exercise. Men on ADT often gain weight and at the same time experience a decrease in muscle mass, bone density, strength, and overall energy levels. These can contribute to a decreased sense of well-being and quality of life. These side effects persist throughout the course of ADT, which may be for many years, and they often continue after ADT is discontinued. *Regular exercise is the single most important lifestyle factor* that can minimize the negative effects of ADT and help to maintain or recover overall quality of life.

Men on ADT gain numerous health benefits from exercising, no matter what type of exercise is performed. In addition to the positive physical effects of exercising, there are other positive effects on psychological well-being, including reducing fatigue and the risk of depression. Exercise may even help to preserve some libido.

> **I should have worked against the fatigue by making a daily practice of some type of active exercise, be it a daily, long walk, routine stretching, and loosening exercises, and so on, but at least something planned. I only continued the routine of most retired men with my only exercise being work around the house, shopping, and the like. I believe that a regular exercise plan and the right mental outlook can counter the effects of fatigue and of muscle loss.**
> **—Charles (Chuck) Maack, prostate cancer survivor and patient advocate**

Exercising Safely

There are several things to consider before beginning an exercise program to ensure that it is undertaken safely and effectively. Here are general safety guidelines that pertain to most endurance exercise (also known as aerobic or cardiovascular exercise) and resistance training (also known as weight lifting):

- Discuss your exercise intentions, goals, and plan with your doctor.
- If you're new to exercise or not sure about how ADT might impact your ability to exercise, ask a qualified exercise professional (QEP) to show you how to safely perform the exercises you plan to do.
- Exercise with a friend or partner to assist you if needed.
- Train in comfortable clothing: running shoes, shorts or track pants, a T-shirt, or moisture-wicking or dry-fit clothes that will keep you cool and dry.
- Protective equipment, such as a helmet, should be worn during any activity that could result in a collision or fall such as riding a bicycle, skiing, or skating.
- Remember to consume water before and during your exercise so you do not get dehydrated.
- Some muscle soreness around 48 hours after a workout is normal especially if you're just starting to exercise. Pain in your joints is not normal and can be a sign of injury. If you are experiencing pain or soreness that lasts longer than 3 to 4 days, see your doctor.

Qualifications and training for qualified exercise professionals (QEPs) working with prostate cancer patients typically include:

- An undergraduate degree in exercise science (e.g., a Bachelor of Kinesiology).
- Certification as an exercise physiologist in good standing with an organization like the American College of Sports Medicine or the Canadian Society for Exercise Physiology.
- Additional certifications specific to exercise and cancer including those offered by the American College of Sports Medicine or other organizations like the University of Northern Colorado Cancer Rehabilitation Institute and Thrive Health Services.
- Minimum of 2 years of experience providing physical activity information, guidance (e.g., exercise prescription), and health screening for older adults as well as individuals living with chronic medical conditions (preferably cancer).
- Work experience in physical activity related to education and behavioral counseling, specifically experience in lifestyle counseling.
- Experience in applied research and critical appraisal of health literature.

Caution

The goal of exercise in the context of ADT is to maintain or improve your physical fitness and psychological well-being. Do not be discouraged if you do not readily see fitness improvements or if you still experience some weight gain despite regular exercise—exercise is still having an important effect at reducing the adverse effects of ADT. In fact, one study conducted by our colleagues demonstrated that men on ADT who were exercising still showed muscle mass loss, but it was much slower compared to men on ADT who were not exercising. It's important to persist with your exercise! Similarly, many men on ADT get discouraged when they either cannot perform at the level they did previously or they expect to be able to achieve. Men who were fit before ADT seem to be at the highest risk for discouragement. Take the necessary precautions for exercise in the body you have now—not in the body you had when you were younger or in the body you might hope to have after significant training.

Some side effects of ADT put patients at increased risk of cardiovascular disease and diabetes. These risks increase with the addition of chemotherapy to your treatment regimen. If you are experiencing other medical conditions, more tailored exercise considerations may be necessary and can be advised on by a QEP. In general, a well-balanced exercise program to address the specific side effects of ADT, as well as many other chronic conditions, should include the following:

- Warm-up exercises to prepare your body for more rigorous activity and prevent injury.
- Aerobic exercise to achieve or maintain a healthy weight and cardiovascular fitness levels.
- Resistance training to improve muscle strength and functional fitness.
- Weight-bearing and balance activities to maintain bone health and prevent fall-related fractures.
- Stretching to increase flexibility and prevent injury.

Warm-Up Exercises

A warm-up is a brief period of activity at a lower intensity than is typically achieved during the main portion of the workout. The warm-up is intended to prepare the body for more vigorous activity and reduce the risk of an injury. Commonly, warm-up exercises resemble those used in the main activity (i.e., incorporating the same muscles) and can become progressively more intense until the exercise intensity zone of the main workout has been achieved. In terms of intensity, you should not be breathing so hard that you cannot easily maintain a conversation during your warm-up.

Always start your training session by warming up for a few minutes. For example, start your session with stretching and a low-intensity cardiovascular exercise. Consider the following:

- Slow walking or marching slowly in place.
- Gentle movements, such as rotating the legs, arms, lower back, and head and neck in circles.
- Light intensity activity on an exercise bike.

Aerobic Exercises

Aerobic training, also known as "cardio" training, improves stamina, which is the ability to sustain repeated movements for long durations. As previously mentioned, men receiving ADT are at a higher risk of developing cardiovascular disease, obesity, and diabetes; thus, a "heart healthy" diet and exercise program is highly recommended. Thirty minutes of aerobic exercises on most days of the week is recommended as a key component of maintaining healthy heart and lung function, and reduces the risk of these conditions. If one continuous bout of 30 minutes of exercise is difficult to fit in your schedule or if you are not quite ready for that duration, you may divide up the time such as accruing three periods of 10 minutes per day to achieve your 30-minute target. Moderations to exercise intensity, like this, may be particularly important if you are on chemotherapy or currently undergoing **radiation therapy** and you are experiencing additional fatigue from these treatments. You do not want to overdo it and then pay the price as your body takes extra time to recover from over-exerting yourself. Start out with exercising for however long you are able, and if you are not on chemotherapy or currently undergoing radiation, you can add additional challenge by adding an additional 5 minutes to your workouts every week or so. Gradually increase the duration of your cardiovascular exercises up to 30 minutes. Then, increase the intensity of the exercise.

The intensity of an exercise program is how hard you are working during the exercise. Some exercise programs suggest a specific target heart rate when you are exercising. There are ways to calculate target heart rate based on your age and general health status. For men in general, the maximal heart rate is calculated as 220 minus your age, and a target heart rate usually falls somewhere between 65% and 90% of that maximal heart rate.

If you have questions about your optimal target heart rate, it is a good idea to talk to your doctor or a QEP. There are other easy ways to monitor your intensity as you exercise. One simple rule-of-thumb is that a moderate intensity exercise should be hard enough to make you sweat. Another simple way of monitoring your intensity is using the Rating of Perceived Exertion (RPE) Scale. The RPE scale is from 0 to 10 where 0 refers to no exertion at all and 10 refers to all-out effort. A moderate intensity on the RPE scale is about 3 to 6 on the 10-point scale.

0	Nothing at all	
0.5	Extremely mild	
1	Very mild	
2	Mild	
3	Moderate	
4		
5	Moderately Vigorous	
6		
7	Vigorous	
8		
9		
10	Maximal exertion	

Source: Modified Borg Scale; Borg, G.A. (1982). Psychophysical bases of perceived exertion. *Medicine & Science in Sports & Exercise*, 14(5), 377–381. Retrieved from https://journals.lww.com/acsm-msse/pages/articleviewer.aspx?year=1982&issue=05000&article=00012&type=abstract

Lastly, a useful technique to determine the intensity of your workout is the "talk test." If, when you are exercising, you are breathing hard enough to make it difficult to talk, then you are likely exercising at a vigorous intensity. Low- to moderate-intensity activity does not typically interrupt normal speech, so strive for an intensity that approaches this threshold of the "talk test." Speech may be a bit interrupted or slower, but you should still be able to talk to some degree. It is important to remember that although you may start breathing heavier during exercise, you should not feel "out of breath."

Here are some aerobic exercises that can be done in the moderate-to-vigorous zone:

- Brisk walking (e.g., walking the dog) or running
- Mall walking in the winter
- Stair climbing (*Note*: Going down stairs can be a little harder on your joints than going up them. If you enjoy climbing stairs, you may want to consider going up one or more flights of stairs and taking the elevator or escalator down.)
- Aqua fitness
- Dance
- Rowing
- Skating
- Cycling (on either a stationary bike or a road bike)

Also, note that there have been studies done comparing normal walking and brisk walking (i.e., low vs. moderate intensity). Results strongly suggest that the health benefits are much greater with brisk walking.

Remember, the goal is eventually to achieve at least 150 minutes of moderate-to-vigorous exercise each week. In many cases, you can listen to music or even watch television while exercising to make the experience more enjoyable. Also consider using a physical activity tracker or pedometer while you exercise. These devices detect steps or movement so that you can keep track of your activity from week-to-week. They can be clipped to your belt or waistband, worn on your wrist, or built into your smartphone. Using activity trackers will allow you to observe your progress, challenge yourself, and perhaps challenge your friends and family!

A comment on high-intensity aerobic exercise: A growing body of scientific literature has examined the role of high-intensity aerobic exercise in people with cancer (usually at close to your maximum heart rate or 9–10/10 on the Borg Scale). Specifically, high-intensity exercise has been tested using a method called interval training, that is, interspersing short bouts of high-intensity exercise with similar durations of rest or light activity. Although the early findings appear promising in terms of improving fitness, more research is required to confirm the safety and applicability to different populations—especially those with cancer. High-intensity interval training, also known as HIIT, should only be performed under the supervision and guidance of a QEP and discussed with your doctor before starting.

Emerging evidence describes that short bursts of high-intensity exercise interspersed with light exercise or rest, known as high-intensity interval training, can be safely performed and provide numerous benefits for people with cancer. Talk to your doctor and a QEP if this type of exercise interests you.

Resistance Training

Resistance training, also known as *strength training* or *weight lifting*, helps build strong, healthy muscles. Safety is a major concern and you should consult with a QEP before starting a resistance training program, as proper form and technique is essential to ensure you do not hurt yourself with repetitive incorrect practice. Resistance training can occur in a variety of ways both with and without equipment.

Since ADT can significantly reduce muscle mass and strength, it is very important that men integrate resistance training into their exercise routine. For many exercises, the resistance of your body weight may be enough, whereas for others it may be beneficial to use free weights or elastic bands. To determine a good workload, aim for the 10 to 12 repetition (rep) range. The first repetitions should be done quite easily. The last ones (11th and 12th) should be difficult but not impossible. When you are able to do 12 repetitions easily, try adding three more repetitions or another set of 12 before increasing the resistance. When the last two reps become more easy, you can then consider increasing the amount of weight. Exercise guidelines for people with cancer recommend resistance training at least three times per week.

A well-rounded resistance exercise program should work all the major muscles of the body, including those in the following table.

Body Regions and Muscle Group	Exercise Examples
Upper Body	
Pectorals	Push-ups, chest/bench press, dumbbell flies
Shoulders	Shoulder press (overhead)[a], lateral (from the sides to the front) or anterior (straight forward) raises
Abdominals	Curl-up, plank, exercise-ball crunches
Biceps	Arm curls with resistance bands or dumbbells
Triceps	Arm extension with resistance bands or dumbbells, dips
Lower Body	
Buttocks	Lunges, stair climbing
Quadriceps	Squats, leg extensions
Calves	Calf raises, toe press
Hamstrings	Leg curls on a machine or using a stability ball

[a]Overhead exercises should be avoided if you have high blood pressure.

Resistance bands, free weights (e.g., barbells, dumbbells), and weight-lifting machines are often used for this type of training but are not absolutely necessary. Exercises such as push-ups, leg raises, and abdominal crunches are also useful at building muscle and strength. Having the correct posture and form during resistance training is very important in order to prevent injuries. If you are new to these types of exercises, we recommend that you review your exercise program with a QEP.

You can prevent unnecessary and potentially dangerous increases in blood pressure if you breathe properly during your resistance training exercises. Breathing out (exhaling) should occur during the "work" phase of the exercise (i.e., the lifting phase), while breathing in (inhaling) should occur during the "relaxing" phase of the exercise (i.e., the lowering or recovery phase). Proper breathing follows a simple four-count pattern: lift—count 1, 2—and lower—count 1, 2. Avoid holding your breath while exercising and try to maintain a steady breathing rhythm.

Keeping Your Bones Healthy

ADT can reduce bone strength, making bones more susceptible to fracture. Two approaches are generally pursued when trying to prevent a fracture: (a) improve bone health and (b) reduce the risk of falls. To achieve these, a comprehensive exercise program should include weight-bearing activities, which promote bone strength, as well as balance exercises to prevent falls.

Weight-bearing activities promote bone maintenance and development. They include any activity that involves being upright and supporting your weight with your legs. The most common weight-bearing activities are

- Walking and running
- Golf, squash, and tennis
- Skipping

One of the most important benefits of a regular exercise program is the maintenance of good balance, which reduces the risk of falls. Your exercise program could incorporate activities specifically designed to maintain and improve balance such as

- Walking on a line (heel to toe) or on your toes
- Balancing on one foot
- Walking backward or sideways
- Tai chi or yoga

Note: These exercises do put you at a risk of a fall; therefore, they should first be attempted near a chair or railing that you can hold on to if you start to fall.

Yoga and Tai Chi

Yoga is an ancient, Eastern mind–body practice. Yoga trains the body and the mind to work together in integrated well-being. Yoga includes a series of poses or physical postures (known as asanas), breathing techniques (known as pranayama), and positive affirmations or meditation to collectively support physical and mental strength and resilience. Yoga has become a popular strategy to manage the physical and the psychological challenges of cancer with many studies demonstrating benefits during and after cancer treatment, such as reducing fatigue, hot flashes, and stress, in addition to improving flexibility, strength, and mood. Yoga can be adapted for various fitness levels, being quite gentle or quite vigorous.

Another Eastern mind–body practice is tai chi. Tai chi comprises a series of slow, rhythmic movements combined with breath and body awareness, meditation, and visualization to foster relaxation and mental health. Tai chi is formally considered a martial art, although commonly practiced for health and wellness. Research has shown that tai chi can reduce blood pressure, stress, and pain, as well as improve mood and physical function.

Yoga and tai chi are considered gentle, low-intensity exercises and thus safe for most patients with cancer. However, if you practice in an inappropriate way, without taking into consideration your current fitness and health history, there is a risk of injury. Certified yoga and tai chi instructors can assist with adapting their intensity and sequences to meet your physical and mental condition.

Cool Down

You should not exercise and then come to a full stop and sit on the couch—after your workout, give your body a few minutes to cool down, to let it gradually come back to resting state. After your exercises, take some time to slowly dial back the intensity, such as slowing the pace of cycling or taking a few minutes for a light walk. In addition to winding down the activity, you can take advantage of this time to do some stretching. We recommend that you maintain a stretch position for a maximum of 20 to 30 seconds. You should feel a slight discomfort when stretching, but not pain. Repeat each stretch a couple of times and make sure you stretch both sides of your body equally. Breathe normally without holding your breath. Each stretching movement should be done slowly and gently, and without bouncing.

Making the Decision to Exercise

Habit and Reason

A useful tool to help you make the decision to exercise is the Pros/Cons table found on page 50. The table is designed to help you recognize motivations for making changes, but also to increase awareness of the reasons why you may be hesitant to change. Filling in this table can help you to identify barriers that may get in the way of you making changes. Recognizing barriers is the first step to overcoming them.

You have an excellent reason, or a "strong pro," to include exercise in your daily routine, and that is managing the possible side effects of ADT! The problem with changing our exercise habits or beginning new ones is that in most cases our physical activity and exercise levels have remained similar for many years and have become cemented in routine and habit. Without thinking about it, we drive to work, we take the elevator, and we sit in front of screens (TVs and computers) for many hours each day. And we "accept" that our days are too full for much else. This behavior, termed the "mechanics of habit," needs to be interrupted or broken. One effective way to do this is to examine your reasons for letting everything else in your day take precedent over exercise and your overall health. Examining these reasons and questioning their validity will sharpen your awareness of sedentary routines and help you break free of habits that may undermine good intentions for exercise.

We recommend *23 and ½ Hours: What Is the Single Best Thing We Can Do for Our Health?* (www.youtube.com/watch?v=aUaInS6HIGo). As the video suggests, limit your daily activities (work, sleep, TV, etc.) to 23½ hours a day and use the remaining half hour to exercise.

Activity: Pros/Cons Table

Your strong reason for exercising—managing the side effects of ADT—is likely one of the things you would list in the pros column of a Pros/Cons table. We will always have reasons both for and against making a change in our behavior. This specific pro gives you a head start in overcoming the cons, so start by placing it at the top of your pros list. Be honest with yourself and spend the same time and energy working on the cons as you do on the pros.

Example:

	PROS	CONS
MAKING THE CHANGE: Exercising	• Reduce the amount of weight I might gain • Prevent loss of physical stamina • Manage fatigue	• Requires significant planning and effort • I will have to reprioritize my schedule to find time to exercise
STAYING THE SAME: Not exercising	• Easier to just carry on the way I am	• My fatigue may continue to get worse • I won't have the fitness to enjoy activities with my family and friends

Try it for yourself. There is an additional blank copy of this table in the Appendix on page 161

	PROS	CONS
MAKING THE CHANGE:		
STAYING THE SAME:		

This planning may sound tedious, but it works. The more the pros outweigh the cons, the stronger your reasons to exercise, which translates into making exercise relevant for you. If you find a lot of reasons in your cons list, you may wish to consider another method of achieving your goal or selecting a different goal to stay physically active.

After you have recorded your pros and cons, see which column has more responses. If your pros of exercising are stronger than your cons, or if there are more of them, then you have demonstrated that a healthy exercise change is worth it. Keep this list handy while you embark on the next step—starting your exercise program.

Setting Goals That Are SMART for You

In addition to having good reasons to exercise, having targets or goals that you wish to achieve, which relate to how you want to feel and what you want to be able to do, can be very motivating. Goal setting also requires some thought to make them valuable to an exercise program. Good goals are SMART goals!

A SMART goal should be

Specific: Describe exactly what it is that you want to achieve. For example, maybe you want to be able to walk the golf course rather than taking the cart; or maybe you want to be able to do 10 push-ups. These goals are specific and will better support your behavior than simply stating you want to be able to walk more or be stronger.

Measurable: You should be able to clearly identify when you have met the goal or how far away you are from achieving the goal. Simply stating that you want to "feel better" is not easily measurable. However, being able to complete your daily chores within 30 minutes or being able to lift 20 pounds. weights are more objective criteria for success and, as measurable goals, you can determine your progress toward meeting them.

Attainable: Your goals should be realistic to achieve. If you set a goal that is too difficult, it can be discouraging to not achieve it. More importantly, the goal will seem so far away that it may lose relevance to you. Make sure your goals are challenging, but within your capacity with an honest effort.

Relevant: If what you are trying to accomplish is not important to you, then it's hard to find the motivation to work toward it. Relevant goals have personal meaning and are worth putting in the necessary efforts and energy to achieve them.

Time-bound: Goals cannot be set with an indefinite period of time. Good goals have a time frame around them to support ongoing action toward achieving them. If your goal is to be able to finish a 2-kilometer hike, set the time frame to allow for your training and an opportunity to achieve it. However, you can set short -and long-term goals.

Example SMART Goals

- By the end of the season, I want to be able to play nine holes of golf while walking the course in under 2 hours.
- I want to be able to hold my abdominal plank for 30 seconds at the end of my 4-week exercise program.
- In 2 months, I want to be able to walk my grandchild around the local park without needing to take a rest break halfway through.

What Are Your SMART Goals?

SMART Goal #1 (try for something in the next 2 to 3 weeks): _____

_____

SMART Goal #2 (try for something in the next 2 months): _____

_____

SMART Goal #3 (try for something in the next 6 to 12 months): _____

_____

Activity: Matching Meaning and Change Using Self-Statements

Changing behavior is a challenge. We are forced to ignore old comfortable patterns of behavior and embrace new, less familiar ones. For men on ADT, a lot of change can be happening at once and adding a new lifestyle behavior may seem overwhelming. People face behavioral changes, like incorporating exercise to a routine, on a moment-by-moment, situation-by-situation basis. This step-by-step process is necessary in the gentle acquisition of change. However, in the early stages of change, people can lose track of why they decided to change in the first place. In their daily "struggles," the meaning of the change can be lost. Ironically, your reasons for initiating change are probably more important early in the change process than at any other time.

A simple method of maintaining your awareness of why you decided to change is the use of "self-statements." Consider the Pros/Cons table you completed in Chapter 2 (p. 34). Write down your most meaningful pros in the following lines. These are your "meaning self-statements." If you ever feel that things are not progressing as quickly as you want, or you feel that you are slipping, read these self-statements to reinforce the meaning of your change.

Meaning Self-Statements:

1. _____

_____

_____

2. _____
   _____
   _____

3. _____
   _____
   _____

Preparing to Successfully Begin Exercising

Thinking about exercise is the first essential step, but thinking is not doing. Are you ready to move from thinking about it to actively planning for it? Thorough preparation is a key to successfully begin exercising. These questions will assist you in developing your Action Plan describing when, where, and with whom you plan to exercise, and what type of exercise(s) you will perform.

Your Action Plan

It is important to choose exercise activities that you believe will benefit your health (i.e., exercises you have confidence in) and that you believe you can maintain over time (i.e., exercises that you have confidence you can perform). There are a wide variety of exercises available to choose from, so take your time. You may want to test out different ones to see which exercises suit you best. To successfully challenge the effects of ADT, choose an exercise or two from each of the exercise categories: warm-up, aerobic, resistance, and weight-bearing.

When Do You Plan to Do It:

- A time free of stress?
- A time when you can put out some extra effort?
- A time when you will have the support you need?

Which days of the week work best for you? _____

What time of the day is most suitable for you? _____

How long do you want to exercise during each session? _____

Remember: You should allow specific muscle groups 48 hours of rest in between each resistance workout to ensure proper recovery. Also, remember to wait at least 1 hour after a heavy meal before exercising.

Where Do You Plan to Do It:

- Inside or outside? Adapt your program to the season.
    - *Inside*—in your home, at a gym, in a "rehab" center or hospital, or in a peer support community center. Remember, you can also do many

exercises in your home with a few inexpensive pieces of equipment such as resistance bands and a stability or exercise ball.
- *Outside*—in a park, on a cycling trail, at a resort or club, or a walking/running circuit in your neighborhood.

Be as specific as possible about where you plan to exercise:

_____

_____

Who Might You Do It With:

- Usually teaming up with someone helps with sticking to a program. By holding each other accountable, you will both benefit from increased exercise.
- If you have a partner, start with that individual. There are few better ways to ensure ongoing success than engaging your partner in exercising with you.
- Talk to your friends and neighbors to find out what type of exercise they do and see if you can join them.
- You might find a great QEP or group fitness class leader that you really connect with and enjoy. Harness that fun experience and stay engaged with your exercise coach.
- Is there a cancer-specific exercise group that you can join?_____

_____

- Sometimes having the support of others going through a similar experience can be very positive.
- Who do you plan to exercise with? Or are you better off exercising on your own?_____

_____

Activity: Action Plan

Much of the information gathered in the previous pages (what, where, when, with whom) can be summarized using an Action Plan. See the following for an example. Remember that it is best to start small with something manageable (e.g., go to the gym twice a week) before you take on larger scale goals (e.g., go to the gym every day).

Action Plan Example: Start Walking Routinely

What I plan to do (My SMART Goal): walk for 15 minutes or more, three times a week for 4 consecutive weeks...starting next week!

When I plan to do it: Monday, Wednesday, and Friday after work

Who I might do it with: with my partner and/or with my dog

Where I plan to do it: around my neighborhood

Why my plan is important: to help control my health risks and reduce fatigue

What might get in the way: poor weather

How I will address what might get in the way: I will go to the mall to walk if the weather is bad

Try it yourself. An additional copy is located in the Appendix on page 162. It helps to be as specific as possible when you are making your Action Plan.

Action Plan/My SMART Goal: _____

What I plan to do: _____

When I plan to do it: _____

Who I might do it with: _____

Where I plan to do it: _____

Why my plan is important: _____

What might get in the way: _____

How I will address what might get in the way: _____

Hang your Action Plan somewhere where you will see it every day, like next to your bathroom mirror, to remind yourself of your commitment to exercise.

Activity: Goal Setting and Confidence

You have identified what type of exercise(s) you plan to do. Now, in order to support your goal, it can be helpful to ask yourself how confident you are that you can be successful in making this change. First, write down your goal.

SMART Exercise Goal 1: _____

(Suggestion: Try an aerobic exercise goal!)

i) Rate how confident you feel that you'll achieve your exercise goal:
   1   2   3   4   5   6   7   8   9   10
   Not confident   Very confident

ii) Rate how motivated you are to accomplish your exercise goal:
   1   2   3   4   5   6   7   8   9   10
   Not motivated   Very motivated

iii) Rate how likely you are to actually carry out your exercise goal:
   1   2   3   4   5   6   7   8   9   10
   Not likely   Very likely

SMART Exercise Goal 2: _____

(Suggestion: Try a resistance training goal!)

i) Rate how confident you feel that you'll achieve your exercise goal:
   1   2   3   4   5   6   7   8   9   10
   Not confident   Very confident

ii) Rate how motivated you are to accomplish your exercise goal:
   1   2   3   4   5   6   7   8   9   10
   Not motivated   Very motivated

iii) Rate how likely you are to actually carry out your exercise goal:
   1   2   3   4   5   6   7   8   9   10
   Not likely   Very likely

A note about confidence—it counts! Behavioral science research has determined that one's level of confidence in embarking on a health-related change is the strongest predictor of success.

- Any exercise recommendation that you choose with a confidence rating of less than 7 out of 10 may become the Achilles' heel of an otherwise good Action Plan. Knowing this can help you realize the extra attention and effort that a particular exercise recommendation may require. We suggest that you do not take on more than two recommendations with a confidence rating lower than 7.
- If your motivation level is low, it may be a good time to go back and reexamine what you put in the Pros/Cons table.
- If you do not think you are likely to carry out your exercise goal, it may be better to select a different goal, one that you are more likely to carry out. Small successes can act as momentum, whereas aiming too high can act as

a roadblock. Start small with goals that you are confident you can achieve. For example, start taking the stairs instead of the elevator, or stand up and do some stretching every 30 minutes during your workday.

Maintaining Your Motivation

You have made your change and are exercising regularly. Congratulations! You may be finding your new exercise routine to be no big deal or still a challenge. Either way, you have taken an important step. Getting to the point of exercising regularly is a long and difficult process, and you have done it. This section offers some tips to help you maintain your exercise regimen once you have started.

Managing Lapses and Relapses

A lapse differs from a relapse in both *frequency* and *duration*. A *lapse* is a single instance of failing to stick to your exercise plan; a *relapse* is a series of lapses in succession. Lapses last only as long as it takes to deviate from your exercise plan, for example, the time it takes to miss a planned exercise session. Relapses are lapses repeated and prolonged, that is, missing exercise sessions again and again, sometimes for a short duration (e.g., 1 week while on vacation), but usually over much longer periods.

Most people experience lapses and relapses when they try to make significant lifestyle changes such as maintaining an exercise program. They are a normal and expected part of real life. How those lapses are managed determines how seriously they threaten long-term change. You will very likely experience a lapse or relapse at some point; just remember that exercising regularly is a step-by-step, day-by-day process. You can easily miss a step or two, or day or two, and lose enthusiasm. The key is to turn around the lapse or relapse quickly by restarting your program as soon as possible. A lapse or relapse is a slip, and a slip is not failure. Decisive action and careful planning have enabled you to build a foundation for exercising. Upon a lapse or relapse, we suggest you return to this foundation and review your reasons and plans for exercising (the Pros/Cons table), as well as your methods for handling hard times. Use this reexamination to challenge the lapse or relapse. Managing these temporary setbacks is not that different from making the original commitment to change. But remember, the longer the relapse, the more vulnerable your commitment to exercise.

Reward Yourself

Rewarding yourself is an art. So do it artfully. Try to reward yourself consistently. Do not worry about being too conventional and do not wait until the victory is won. Rewarding yourself amid the struggle is more important. During the first 2 weeks of exercising, try rewarding yourself a little each day. A good reward might be sleeping in an extra 10 minutes, new exercise apparel, some new music to listen to while you exercise, watching a movie, or making time to meet with friends. It does not have to take long and it need not be expensive. Choose a reward that inspires you to exercise and it can help you stay on track.

Some rewards, however, can actually deter you from your overall fitness goals. Often food is used as a reward. It is okay to treat yourself with a "not-so-healthy-snack"—occasionally! If having a food reward encourages you to exercise, then it's a great idea. Regardless of the calorie count, you are exercising and still improving cardiovascular fitness! It may be a helpful point of awareness to think about it this way: A small bag (1.69 oz package; 1.7 oz = ~48 g) of M&M's is a nice reward; however, it is 240 calories. If you want to balance your calorie intake, 30 minutes on the treadmill will burn off those calories.

Another "reward" that is often implemented is a decrease in nonexercise physical activity. For example, if you had a great workout, you might feel like avoiding the stairs that you usually take to your apartment or office. By avoiding these other daily activities you are simply trading one healthy behavior for another, resulting in less net benefit. Try to maintain your daily, nonexercise physical activities. Compensating for healthy behaviors with unhealthy ones too frequently can undermine your progress. So, again, give yourself a treat when you have done a good job with your exercise, but too many treats (or the wrong treats) may in fact set you back.

Support

Research has shown that social support contributes to healthy lifestyle changes. In study after study, support has made a major difference in successful exercising, especially if your spouse/partner or a close friend is also participating in exercising. A joint effort to exercise regularly promotes mutual encouragement.

Providing support to your significant other for exercise may be the best support you can provide.

The key ingredients of "precise support" are threefold:

- *Timing*: It must be there *when* a person needs it.
- *Focus*: It must be focused *where* a person needs it—emotionally, practically, and so on.
- *Expression*: It must be expressed in the specific way that best motivates the individual to achieve his or her goal.

Activity: Identifying and Overcoming Barriers to Starting and Maintaining an Exercise Program

I feel too tired. When we feel fatigued our instinct is to rest. Those who are struggling with fatigue may worry that they will not have the energy to do their usual activities if they spend energy exercising. You do need to rest, but resting too much can lead to further deconditioning, which will in turn lead to more fatigue.

I do not have the willpower. You *do* have the willpower; you simply need to find a way to unleash this power! You are prepared. You have the main ingredients to a successful exercise program. Consider this: How often do you dread the thought of doing something you enjoy? Probably, quite rarely (or never). So if you can find the fun in your activity, it will ensure that your willpower can be realized. Think of ways to integrate things you enjoy while exercising, like music, your friends/family, a television show, or an environment that is relaxing (e.g., a park) or stimulating (e.g., a gym) for you.

It is not the right time. There is no perfect time. Now may be as good a time as any. There will always be some stress in your life. There will always be distractions. You can make progress now.

My life is not going well. This little change is not going to make a difference. Just the opposite. You have got to start somewhere and sometimes you need a little self-compassion to take the pressure off. Exercise can really help—it's worth giving it a try!

I have aches and pains that limit how I exercise. We all have certain aches and pains that make some exercises uncomfortable or possibly painful. It's important to avoid exercises that cause pain. For any aches and pains that you have that may limit your activities, consider alternate forms of exercise. For example, if walking bothers your knees, try cycling, swimming, or using an elliptical machine. A QEP can help adjust your exercise program to accommodate any discomforts. If the pain persists when you are not exercising, you should consult your physician.

Other barriers and ways to address or challenge those barriers:

_____

_____

_____

Exercise: Essentials

Getting physical exercise is arguably the most important thing you can do to manage ADT side effects. Men on ADT often gain weight as fat, at the same time experiencing a decrease in muscle mass, bone density, strength, and overall energy levels. Exercise can help manage all of these side effects.

We discussed the rationale for beginning an exercise program and gave recommendations for creating one that works best for you. We also acknowledged that maintaining an exercise program over the long term can be difficult and provided tips on making exercise safe and enjoyable, as well as strategies that will help you overcome challenges that may arise.

Successful change lies in decision-making, planning, initiating, trial and error, and revising goals as necessary—all leading to confidence in maintaining a new lifestyle. As you continue your journey toward a life with regular exercise as a routine, increased confidence will lead to an increase in your success, overcoming lapses and relapses quickly. In time, this feedback loop from action to confidence to action again will result in successfully integrating exercise into your everyday life. Incorporating regular exercise into your daily routine is likely to be the single most important thing you do to maintain a good quality of life while on ADT.

Moving Forward: Questions for Discussion

- What exercise do I enjoy most?
- Who would I enjoy exercising with?
- What are the three most important reasons for me to exercise?
- What time of the day would I feel most comfortable and motivated to exercise?
- What lingering aches and pains do I have?
- How will I adapt my exercises to prevent them from being aggravated?
- What equipment or supplies do I require to exercise effectively, and where can I access them?
- What barriers to exercise can I anticipate encountering as I work toward maintaining a routine exercise program? How will I address them?
- What three specific goals do I hope to accomplish at the end of 6 weeks of exercise?
- How will I reward myself for exercising?

NOTES:

_____

_____

_____

_____

_____

_____

Exercise

4

HEALTHY EATING

A well-balanced diet can help manage several androgen deprivation therapy (ADT) side effects. There are some general principles, though, about diet and cancer that one should be aware of. The first one is that a diet, which may help prevent a cancer from occurring in the first place, is not likely to cure cancer once cancer has been diagnosed. This is true for prostate cancer. At the moment, there is no food or supplement that has been shown to cure prostate cancer. However, being on a diet that can help to prevent cancer, even if one already has prostate cancer, makes sense as it can help protect you from getting another type of cancer. Perhaps the best reason to eat healthy is to reduce the risk of cardiovascular disease, which is a major killer of men with prostate cancer.

A second general principle when it comes to diet is that moderation is always in order. If a certain amount of a food is good for your health, it does not necessarily follow that twice as much of that food will make you twice as healthy. In fact, many things that we consume, which may be good for us at one serving or dose, may be harmful if taken excessively. A good example of this—discussed under the subheading, "Calcium"— is taking calcium. Calcium and vitamin D work together to help keep one's bones strong while on ADT, but too much calcium can lead to new health problems, such as kidney stones. For any food or supplement you ingest, it is best to stay within the most up-to-date guidelines.

When you are on ADT, you may experience common side effects such as a loss of muscle mass and weight gained as fat mainly at your waistline. Men treated with ADT are also at increased risk of osteoporosis, diabetes, and cardiovascular problems. Over time, ADT causes decrease in bone mineral density, increased body weight, poor blood sugar regulation, and raised cholesterol, as well as altered triglycerides that can collectively contribute to more serious health risks. Fortunately, eating healthy can help you manage your weight and reduce these risk factors.

As a general rule, eating healthy involves consuming lots of fruits, vegetables, and lean protein. Eating healthy also means eating fresh food as much as possible. Foods that have been processed often contain high amounts of salt, sugar, preservatives, and unhealthy fats. Processed foods also tend to be lower in nutrition and higher in calories.

RECOMMENDATIONS

- **Eat more high-fiber foods (e.g., whole grains, vegetables, nuts, and fruits).**
- **Eat more lean meat (e.g., fish, chicken rather than beef, pork, and lamb).**
- **Eat less saturated and trans fats.**
- **Limit salt and sugar intake.**
- **Eat less-processed foods.**

Reading Food Labels

Most packaged foods in the United States and Canada have mandatory nutrition labeling. Read the labels carefully and make an effort to eat food with the highest nutritional content. The values on most labels are based on a diet of 2,000 calories per day. Look for foods or beverages high in nutrients such as calcium, vitamin C, vitamin A, thiamin, niacin, and fiber. Also check the amounts of fat (saturated and trans fat), cholesterol, sugar, and sodium—and limit these. Remember to look at the serving size and the total number of calories, and compare this to the portion you actually eat. The Percent Daily Value (%DV) on the Nutrition Facts table provides information on calories and 13 nutrients. This can be used to compare products and make a healthier choice. It helps to know what the recommended daily allowance (RDA) is for each nutrient that is discussed further in the following. A quick rule for using the %DV is that 5% or less is a small amount of a nutrient in an overall day and 20% or higher is a lot for a single food in a day.

> The U.S. Department of Health & Human Services has more information regarding labels, including some helpful graphics. This can be accessed on their website (www.fda.gov) under the "Food" tab.

Fats

Fats from the food you eat have many functions in the body. They provide energy and, when stored as body fat, help to keep your body warm. Fats also provide the building materials for cells and some **hormones**, and they help the body absorb some vitamins. Your body needs fat to function, but moderation is important. Too much fat can be damaging to your health. Eating a high-fat diet increases your risk of obesity and related health problems, such as heart disease and diabetes. Because these are the same health risks men on ADT experience, combining a high-fat diet with ADT will make you more susceptible to these health problems.

Fats are classified into two groups:

1. *Unsaturated fats* are generally considered to be the "healthy" fats. They are categorized as either *monounsaturated* (found in olive and canola oils, avocados, and most nuts) or *polyunsaturated* (found in vegetable oils, meat products, and fish). There are some types of polyunsaturated fats that your body cannot produce, but still needs. These are considered "essential" fatty acids and must be obtained from your diet. Linoleic acid (omega-6; LA) and alpha-linolenic acid (omega-3; ALA) are two polyunsaturated fatty acids that are considered "essential." They should be consumed regularly, but in moderation. To learn more about omega fatty acids, see pages 71 to 73.
2. *Saturated fats* are considered to be the "less healthy" fats. Limit foods high in saturated fats and replace them with foods containing unsaturated fats (see previous). Saturated fats are solid at room temperature. Most of the saturated fats in our diet come from animal products, such as meat and dairy.

Trans fats are a type of unsaturated fat, but they are an exception to the "healthy" rule as they are processed in the body similarly to saturated fats. Trans fats are present naturally in small quantities in foods such as meat and dairy, but in Western diets most trans fats come from processed foods during a process called *hydrogenation*. This process turns oils into semisolid products, including partially hydrogenated oils such as vegetable shortening and some types of margarine. Hydrogenation makes food products last longer, but it also makes trans fats especially harmful. Other foods containing trans fats include potato chips, chocolate bars, and many foods made from or fried in hydrogenated fat. When shopping, it is recommended to read the labels to determine the amount of trans fats in the products you buy, and aim to choose foods with no (or limited) trans fats.

Dietary fats are a part of the building blocks of androgens. There is some evidence that high-fat diets can raise **androgen** levels. For example, vegetarians (who often consume less dietary fat) tend to have lower levels of **testosterone** than meat eaters. One theory under investigation is whether men with prostate cancer may benefit from a diet lower in fat and cholesterol aimed at decreasing testosterone. The goal of reducing testosterone is similar to treatment with ADT, which attempts to "starve" prostate cancer cells of testosterone.

RECOMMENDATIONS

- Aim to eat more fruits and vegetables that are naturally low in fat.
- Focus on quality, also keeping in mind the amount that you eat.
- Choose plant-based fats, such as olive, safflower, canola, or sesame oils, which have greater health benefits.
- Eat smaller (palm-sized) portions of meat, especially red meat.
- When preparing poultry or other meats, remove the skin and trim off excess fat.
- Cut back on fried and processed foods.
- If you fry your meat, remember to drain the fat from the pan before adding sauces.
- Stir-frying, sautéing, baking, or grilling your food are all better options than frying or deep-frying.
- Cut down on butter, margarine, oils, sauces, gravy, and cream.

Practice mindful eating, and be aware of what you are eating. Choose foods with high nutritional value and low fat content when you shop for groceries. Some foods are naturally low in fat such as fruits, vegetables, and most grains. When choosing low-fat foods, some are better in nutritional value than others. Lower fat dairy products are a good choice because only the fat is reduced. However, be mindful that some lower fat foods may replace the fat with sugar, so aim for foods lower in calories.

Pretty soon, making healthier choices will become a habit.

Protein

Our bodies need protein to build tissue for growth and repair. The protein in our diets comes from two sources: animals and plants. Animal sources of protein include meat, fish, poultry, eggs, and dairy products. Red and white meat are protein rich and contribute different nutrients to the diet. Red meats (e.g., beef, pork, lamb) are higher in fat, but also provide benefits like vitamin B_{12} and iron. Despite these benefits, there are a few things you need to consider when planning a healthy diet.

Western diets typically include too much animal protein and not enough vegetables, fruits, and legumes (i.e., peas, beans, lentils). Most cuts of red meat are also high in fat, and most processed meats (e.g., bacon, deli meats) are high in salt, fat, and preservatives. White meat from poultry is typically a better healthy choice compared to red meat. Furthermore, meat cooked at high temperatures that results in charring can burn off protein and form cancer-causing by-products.

Fish is a "heart-healthier" and leaner source of protein than most meat because most types of fish are naturally low in fat, particularly saturated fat.

Choose fish packed in water (rather than oil such as in canned fish) to avoid added fat. Also, frying any type of fish may increase the amount of unhealthy fat. Steaming, broiling, roasting, poaching, and baking are better options.

Milk and dairy products can also be high in fat, particularly saturated fat. When eating dairy or dairy alternatives, it is recommended that you opt for lower fat choices (i.e., skim or 1% dairy milks, almond or soy milk, low-fat cheeses, and yogurts), and look for dairy products that do not have a lot of added sugars.

The following table describes various sources of protein.

Meat or Meat Alternative	Serving Size or Amount
Cooked fish, shellfish, poultry, or lean beef, pork, and lamb	2 1/2 oz (75 g) or 1/2 cup (125 mL) or the size of a deck of playing cards
Cooked beans, peas, lentils, or tofu	3/4 cup (175 mL)
Nuts or seeds (shelled)	1/4 cup (60 mL)
Peanut butter or other nut butters	2 tbsp (30 mL)
Eggs	2 eggs

Based on the *Dietary Reference Intakes for Americans and Canadians*, it is recommended that adults consume 0.8 g of protein per kilogram of body weight. On average that means a daily intake of 46 g of protein for women and 56 g for men.

A strategy for finding the right fat–protein balance is to focus on plant protein. Plants that provide protein are typically rich in vitamins and minerals as well as a source of health-promoting phytonutrients and fiber. Plant foods are also generally low in fat, or the fat is unsaturated. Unlike meat, plant products contain carbohydrates of the "complex" or starchy type (see following table). The richest sources of plant protein are legumes, such as dried peas (e.g., split peas) and beans (e.g., kidney, chickpea).

Include a variety of plant protein sources in your daily diet. The following table gives you an idea of some plant protein sources:

Legumes	Grain	Nuts and Seeds
Soybeans/soy products	Barley	Almonds
Peanuts	Bulgur	Walnuts
Chickpeas	Couscous	Cashews
Lentils	Oats	Chestnuts
Split peas	Rice	Pecans
Kidney beans	Wheat	Pumpkin seeds
Pinto beans	Rye	Sesame seeds
Fava beans		Quinoa

Legumes, nuts, and seeds are the best sources of plant protein. Grains provide a small amount of protein to a diet, particularly for vegetarians. Quinoa, which is sometimes eaten in similar ways to a grain, is actually a seed and is rich in protein.

Plant foods are high in fiber and you may experience gastrointestinal problems if you increase your consumption too quickly. Try introducing plant protein gradually into your diet, and drink water with your meals.

RECOMMENDATIONS

- **Eat a variety of protein-rich foods, including fish, seafood, lean meat and poultry, eggs, beans (such as soy) and peas, and nuts and seeds.**
- **Replace protein-rich foods that are higher in fat, preservatives, and salt with those that are lower in those substances.**
- **Eat fish at least twice a week.**
- **Choose low-fat or fat-free milk and milk products, such as milk, yogurt, and cheese.**

Carbohydrates

Carbohydrates are a source of energy. Although they often get a bad reputation for being "fattening," in reality, carbohydrates have fewer calories (or food energy) per gram than fats (4 calories compared with 9 calories). Carbohydrates are classified as simple or complex, based on the size of the molecules.

Simple carbohydrates are sugars and can be monosaccharides (glucose, fructose, galactose) or disaccharides (maltose, sucrose, lactose). They are absorbed quickly into the body, raising blood sugar, and are considered "fast" energy. Foods such as honey, molasses, white sugar, brown sugar, raw sugar, and maple and corn syrups are similar in nutritional value and high in simple carbohydrates.

Complex carbohydrates are polysaccharides, sometimes called *starches* and *fiber*. Polysaccharides are digested and absorbed slower than simple carbohydrates, but are also eventually broken down into sugars. Starches are present in grains, legumes, and root vegetables (e.g., potatoes and yams).

Fiber is a type of complex carbohydrate. Fiber is found only in plant foods, such as fruits and vegetables, grains, beans other legumes, nuts, and seeds. It is the indigestible part of the plant, and thus it is not digested by the body. Fiber nevertheless has many benefits and assists in the digestion of other foods. Aim for at least 25 grams of fiber daily. Plant foods that are rich in fiber are also a good source of vitamins, minerals, and carbohydrates.

RECOMMENDATIONS

- Eat whole foods rich in complex carbohydrates, such as whole grains, legumes, fruits, and vegetables, as part of a balanced diet.
- Limit "refined" carbohydrates found in starchy and sugary processed foods. The processing lowers their nutritional value. Check the nutrition label and choose foods with at least 2 grams of fiber per serving.
- Limit products with added sugar. They have extra calories without any other nutritional benefit.

Determining Your Current BMI

BMI stands for **body mass index**. This measure is a tool that can help determine if you are presently at a healthy weight for your height—and to assess potential health risks. You can ask your local gym or your family doctor to help you determine your BMI or you can use the following formula. The BMI is a generalization of body type; it does not differentiate fat weight from fat-free weight (muscle or bone), and therefore it has been criticized. If you are not convinced your BMI is an accurate assessment of your health risk, having your body fat percentage and/or waist-to-hip ratio measured may help to better determine your healthy weight range.

If you would like to determine your BMI on your own, you can use the following formulas:

English: BMI = weight in pounds/(height in inches × height in inches) × 703
Metric: BMI = weight in kilograms/(height in meters × height in meters)

Pay special attention to the units in the formula; otherwise, the result will not be accurate. There are also many BMI calculators available online.

Note: For persons 65 years and older, the "normal" range may begin slightly above BMI 18.5 and extend into the "overweight" range. The BMI may underestimate body fat in older persons.

The following table shows the different classifications of BMI and their health risks:

Classification	BMI Category	Risk of Developing Health Problems
Underweight	<18.5	Increased
Normal weight	18.5–24.9	Least
Overweight	25.0–29.9	Increased
Obese	≥30.0	Highest

BMI; body mass index

Along with BMI, measuring your waist circumference can be a good approximation of where you stand in terms of health risks. The larger one's waist circumference is above the population average, the greater are the health risks. In North America, the "cut-off" for what is considered healthy is 40 inches (102 cm) for men and 35 inches (88 cm) for women. Measurements above the recommended BMI range and waist circumference values (particularly if both are elevated) put you at greater risk for developing health problems or worsening existing conditions.

Estimating Your Nutritional Needs

The Dietary Reference Intakes (in Canada and the United States) currently recommend the following percentages for daily calorie intake:

- *Fat*: 20% to 35% (no more than 10% from saturated sources)
- *Protein*: 10% to 35%
- *Carbohydrate*: 45% to 65%

If you decide to change your diet to meet these recommendations, remember that if you are within the healthy weight range, the goal is to maintain your present calorie (energy) intake. To keep your calories balanced, when you add more of certain types of food to your diet (e.g., complex carbohydrates, such as those in whole grain cereals or breads), you will need to decrease calories from other foods (e.g., saturated fats).

To estimate your daily requirements, decide on a realistic goal for the percentage of fat, protein, and carbohydrates you would like to eat from within the recommended ranges. Protein, like carbohydrates, has approximately 4 calories per gram. Fats have 9 calories per gram. Alcohol also contributes calories (about 7 calories per gram), so do not forget to factor it in, if you drink.

Using an estimated calorie goal based on your activity level, you can calculate the grams of fat, protein, and carbohydrates using the following equation:

[(Calories × Percentage of intake)/Calories per gram of carbohydrate, protein, or fat] = Daily grams of carbohydrate, protein, or fat

For example, if you eat about 2,000 calories per day, and you would like to eat 55% of your total calories as carbohydrates, the amount in grams would be calculated as follows:

[(2,000 calories × 0.55)/4 calories per gram] = 275 grams of carbohydrate per day

There is no golden rule to follow when determining your daily calorie intake; it depends on several factors, including your weight, age, sex, and activity level. A typical value for a middle-aged man is about 2,000 to 2,500 calories per day. To estimate your calorie consumption, record what you eat for several days and calculate your average intake. For more precise calculations, consult a dietitian to evaluate your energy requirements.

If you find that you are gaining weight while on ADT, you may need to reduce the number of calories you eat. Remember, if you need to lose weight, for best results you will need to consistently eat less and/or burn off more calories (from physical activity) than your body typically needs in a day. You cannot lose weight if you consume more calories than you burn off.

> **For more information on nutrition and weight management, help on tracking what you eat, an online BMI calculator, and more, visit www.choosemyplate.gov, a website designed by the U.S. Department of Agriculture. The Academy of Nutrition and Dietetics (www.eatright.org) is also an excellent resource. There are also several "apps" available to help you track your food intake and your physical activity.**

Omega-3 Fatty Acids

Omega-3 fatty acids are important for overall health and are found mainly in fish, seafood, some nuts, seeds, and vegetable oils. There are three types of polyunsaturated omega-3 fatty acids: ALA, eicosapentaenoic acid (EPA), and docosahexaenoic acid (DHA). ALA is called an essential fatty acid because it cannot be formed in the body; it must be acquired through your diet. Rich sources are flaxseed, meats, and cereals. ALA can be converted to EPA and DHA in our bodies, but this process is inefficient; therefore, it is best to include foods rich in all three types of omega-3 fatty acids in your diet. EPA and DHA are found in fatty, cold-water fish such as salmon, herring, mackerel, sardines, bass, and white albacore tuna. Fish are recommended as an excellent source of omega-3 fatty acids.

Omega-3 Fatty Acid Supplements

Foods are the preferred way to meet daily needs. Foods have a wide range of other vitamins, minerals, fiber, and anticancer compounds not found in supplements and do not have the same risk of possible adverse effects. Although diets rich in ALA have been shown to reduce heart disease in men, the role of omega-3 fatty acids or fish oil supplements (rich in omega-3) in decreasing prostate cancer progression remains unclear. Men with prostate cancer are recommended to eat fish twice per week and include other foods rich in omega-3 fatty acids as part of their daily diet for general health benefits.

Furthermore, there is no evidence to suggest that men on ADT benefit from omega-3 supplements. Men with a family history of stroke or on blood-thinning medications (including aspirin) could, in rare instances, experience negative side effects from such supplements. If you are thinking of taking a supplement rich in omega-3, you should consult with your physician or a registered dietitian first.

The best food sources of omega-3 include the following:

- Fish and seafood including herring, anchovies, mackerel, sardines, salmon, whitefish, halibut, trout, bass, oysters, Arctic char, cod, tuna, and mussels are high in omega-3.
- Some vegetable oils, including flaxseed and canola oil, are good sources.
- Some other plant foods are a rich source (e.g., some nuts and seeds). The best sources are flaxseed (ground), chia and hemp seeds, walnuts, and soy foods including soybeans, edamame, and tofu. Other nuts, such as pecans, also contain omega-3.

Note: This list includes food sources and not any supplement sources of omega-3 fatty acids such as fish oils.

In addition, some foods are now fortified with omega-3 fats and therefore become good sources. Foods commonly fortified include some brands of milk, soy beverages, yogurt, and eggs. Check the label!

A limited amount of omega-3 fatty acids are found in grains, such as wheat germ. But otherwise, grains and most vegetables and fruit are *not* good sources.

RECOMMENDATIONS

- **Get your omega-3 fatty acids from eating fish and other sources, rather than from taking supplements.**
- **Eating fish even once a week may be enough to reap some positive benefits.**
- **The RDA for omega-3 fatty acids is 1.6 grams for adult males.**

Omega-6 Fatty Acids

LA is a type of essential omega-6 fatty acid and is found in animal fats, nuts, and vegetable oils. It is the most commonly consumed polyunsaturated fatty acid in the Western diet. Because it is so common in popular foods, we often eat more than we need. It is recommended that you try to balance your omega-3 and omega-6 intake by substituting fish for meat at least once a week and choosing oils with less omega-6.

Dietary recommendations for omega-3 and omega-6 are shown in the following table:

Fatty Acid	Age	General Recommended Daily Intake (g)
Omega-3	All ages	1.6[a]
Omega-6	31–50 years	17
	51 and older	14

[a]Up to 10% of daily intake can be consumed as EPA and/or DHA.
DHA, docosahexaenoic acid; EPA, eicosapentaenoic acid.

RECOMMENDATIONS

- **Use olive oil or canola oil instead of safflower, sunflower, or soybean oil.**
- **Remember: A little oil goes a long way.**

Soy

Soybeans and several foods made from soybeans are recommended as part of a healthy diet and may have additional benefits for men with prostate cancer. Soy foods are a great substitute for meat because they are a rich source of protein that is low in saturated fat. Soy foods also contain special compounds called isoflavones, which, among other things, may help reduce the risk of prostate cancer progression and reduce your likelihood of developing osteoporosis or cardiovascular disease. Soy-based foods are becoming more popular and are easy to find in grocery stores—but the nutritional value can vary widely. Soy foods are a healthy choice. However, how beneficial soy is in controlling prostate cancer is still under investigation. Here is a list of common soy foods:

Tofu is a semisoft food made from adding mineral salt to soymilk. It is a convenient and nutritious substitute for meat. Tofu can be purchased at varying degrees of firmness. The softer form is best for sauces and dips; the denser type of tofu (higher in protein) is for grilling, baking, and stir-frying. Tofu lends itself well to a variety of recipes because it absorbs flavors mixed in with it.

Soy beverage is made from ground and cooked soybeans. The soy "milk" is filtered out during this process. It can be used as a dairy substitute. It is the easiest soy food to incorporate, consumed straight from the carton, on breakfast cereal, or used in cooking or baking. Soy beverages with the highest nutritional value are those fortified with calcium and vitamin D (check the label) and those made with whole soybean, rather than extracts such as "soy protein isolates." "Plain" or "original" beverages are also best because they contain fewer added sugars than flavored soy beverages.

Tempeh, a textured vegetable protein (TVP) made from cooked and fermented soybeans, like other soy foods, can also be used as a meat substitute. It is high in calcium, iron, zinc, and fiber and, like all plant foods, is cholesterol free. Another TVP, *miso*, is made from fermented soybean paste and is commonly used in soups. Miso contains a lot of salt, though, so it should not be eaten in large quantities.

Natto, yet another fermented soy product, has a sticky texture and a distinct smell. It is often served on top of rice.

Processed soy foods: Soy powder is available in different flavors, as flour (whole-ground soy flour is best), granules, or the extracted protein (i.e., "isolate"). Among the soy products, defatted soy flour and soy isolates contain the most protein. Soy powder can be mixed with fruit juices, soy beverage, or skim milk. However, overall, soybeans and soy foods that are made from and contain more of the whole soybean offer the greatest nutritional value and are preferred over processed soy foods including soy powders.

Soy sauce and *tamari*: Many types of "soy sauce" are not a good source of soy and typically are made from colored, flavored salt water. To get the real benefit of soy, use tamari, which is a fermented brew made from soybeans.

There are other soy products as well. These include roasted soy "nuts" and steamed soybeans known as edamame. These are typically salted and people should be aware of that if they are trying to keep their salt intake down.

RECOMMENDATIONS

- Soybeans and soy foods made from soybeans are a rich source of protein, and for maximum health benefits, soy can be used as a meat substitute.
- Levels of isoflavones, and the amount of protein, fat, and calcium, can differ widely across brands and forms of soy foods. Read the labels carefully to assess their nutritional value.
- Choose regular or low-fat varieties. If you are drinking soy beverages as a substitute for milk, select brands fortified with calcium and vitamin D.
- Avoid nonfat soy beverages, since soybeans lose some of their beneficial properties when completely defatted.
- Men on protein-restricted diets for medical reasons (e.g., diabetes, liver, or kidney disease) should consult their doctor before adding soy to their diet.
- Adding soy (or any new food) to your diet may cause you to gain a few pounds if there is no reduction in other foods. But soy foods can be used as a substitute for meat and thus can help you to avoid excess animal fat in your diet. Substituting soy for meat can also improve the quality of fat in your diet by adding healthier plant fats.

Vitamin D

Vitamin D increases the body's ability to absorb calcium, which is important for bone health. Emerging research suggests a wider role of vitamin D in human health, including a role in controlling cell growth. Sunlight triggers the body to produce vitamin D, and is the main source of this nutrient. But sunshine does not do this very well for certain populations, such as African American and elderly men, and in areas where sunlight is limited (resulting in low vitamin D levels, at least during the winter period).

At this time, the strongest evidence for vitamin D relates to maintaining bone health. Research into the possible benefits of vitamin D for men with prostate cancer is currently in progress.

How Do I Get Enough Vitamin D?

A primary food source of vitamin D is fatty fish, but North Americans often do not eat enough fish and may get more of their vitamin D from foods with vitamin D added (i.e., fortified foods). In Canada, it is mandatory for vitamin D to be added to milk. Other foods, such as margarine, soy and other plant-based beverages, goat's milk, orange juice, and some cereals may also have vitamin D added. In the United States, most milk is voluntarily fortified with 100 IU of vitamin D per cup. The Dietary Reference Intakes for Canadians and Americans recommend a daily vitamin D intake of 600 IU (up to age 70) and up to 800 IU (over age 70) from all sources. At present, the tolerable upper limit (UL) is considered to be 4,000 IU/day (from all sources). You may have noticed that there is a wide range of recommendations for vitamin D from other organizations. Generally, these recommendations advise from 600 IU up to 2,000 IU per day, but in the last several years the general consensus is that more may be better, provided it remains under the UL. Given this general trend, we recommend closer to 1,500 or 2,000 IU. The role of vitamin D in human health and the optimal amount of vitamin D is an active area of research. At the moment, there is no evidence that patients on ADT benefit substantially from doses above the recommended amounts.

In spring and summer, 15 minutes a day of direct sun exposure without sunscreen in the early morning or late afternoon is adequate for most people to meet the RDA for vitamin D within their own body. With this small amount of exposure, the risk of skin cancer is miniscule.

Finally, as the following table indicates, fish are a good dietary source of vitamin D.

Type of Fish	Vitamin D (IU/100 g)
Atlantic cod	40[a]
Tuna (canned in oil, drained)	236
Sea bass (per fillet)	291.54[a]
Atlantic mackerel	324[a]
Catfish (wild)	450[a]
Pacific sardines (canned in tomato sauce, drained)	480
Greenland halibut	540[a]
Sockeye salmon (canned, drained)	763
Atlantic herring	1,465[a]

[a]IU calculated for cooked fish based on raw weights.

Calcium

Calcium is an important mineral, which helps to build and maintain strong bones. The RDA is 1,000 to 1,200 mg from all sources including regular and fortified foods plus supplements. Despite these benefits, recent studies have found a possible association between *excessive* calcium intake and prostate cancer. As with all nutrients, it is possible to get too much calcium. The UL for calcium is 2,500 mg (<50 years) and 2,000 mg (>50 years). Research has shown that men who consume more than 2,000 mg of calcium per day (from a combination of diet and supplements) experience an elevated risk of advanced and metastatic disease. Another important side effect of too much calcium is the risk of kidney stones. Therefore, it is recommended that consumption stay below the upper tolerable limit, and probably why we see recommendations closer to the 1,000 to 1,200 mg range.

This does not mean that men should stop eating dairy or other calcium-rich foods; calcium intake within the RDA has not been linked to prostate cancer. Men with prostate cancer should try to achieve the RDA through diet; however, if you do not get enough from your food, you may consider supplementation.

Calcium in Your Diet

An adult man (19–70 years old) should consume 1,000 mg of calcium a day. If you are 70 or older you should consume 1,200 mg/day. However, your physician may recommend more than this and we have certainly seen recommendations increasing in recent years, into the range of 1,500 to 2,000 mg since men on ADT taking 1,000 mg may still show bone loss. Some healthcare providers also recommend taking calcium in smaller doses throughout the day (e.g., 500 mg, three times per day, rather than 1,500 mg all at once) to aid in absorption. Getting adequate (but not excessive) calcium is particularly important for men on long-term ADT because of the increased risk of osteoporosis and bone fractures. If you follow the recommendations here, you will likely meet your daily need.

> You can access a useful tool for calculating your calcium intake at Osteoporosis Canada's website (www.osteoporosis.ca/osteoporosis-and-you/nutrition/calculate-my-calcium).

Given that there are risks associated with taking more than the UL of calcium, note how much calcium you are getting in your daily diet, so that you do not take too much. For example, if you are getting 1,000 mg from your food per day, you would not also want to supplement with 1,500 mg or more as that would exceed the RDA. In the table on the following page is a list of foods that you may want to consider integrating more of into your regular diet. Included there are the approximate amounts of calcium in each of these foods. If you wish to consume little or no milk products and want other options for foods rich in calcium, try drinking fortified beverages (i.e., brands with added calcium) or eating calcium-rich vegetables and legumes (e.g., beans, spinach, broccoli). Appropriate portions of these foods (e.g., a cup of cooked broccoli or beans as a side dish) may not be as rich a source of calcium, but do offer some variety to your diet.

For more information on calcium content in foods, visit the website of the Office of Dietary Supplements (National Institutes of Health, ods.od.nih.gov), or you can look up the nutrient information of any food by visiting the U.S. Department of Agriculture website (ndb.nal.usda.gov).

Source of Calcium	**Serving Size**	**Approximate Amount of Calcium (mg)**
Yogurt (plain, low-fat)	1 cup	415
Canned sardines (in oil, including bones)	85 g (3 oz)	325
Cheddar cheese	43 g (1.5 oz)	310
Milk (whole, skim, or low-fat)	1 cup	300
Soy milk (calcium-fortified)	1 cup	300
Orange juice (calcium-fortified)	¾ cup	260
Tofu (firm, made with calcium sulfate)	½ cup	250
Canned salmon (pink, including bones)	85 g (3 oz)	180
Cottage cheese (1% milk fat)	1 cup	140
Kale (raw)	1 cup	100
Frozen yogurt (vanilla, soft serve)	½ cup	100
Sesame seeds (whole, dried)	1 tbsp	88
Broccoli (raw)	1 cup	42
Chick-peas (canned)	½ cup	38
Bread (whole-wheat)	1 slice	30
Sweet potato (baked)	½ cup	30
Cream cheese (regular)	1 tbsp	14

RECOMMENDATIONS

Calcium intake of 1,200 to 1,500 mg daily, preferably from diet (with 1,000–1,500 IU of vitamin D), is recommended for general health and to prevent bone loss and fractures.

Before we leave the subject of vitamin D and calcium, we acknowledge that the data showing that calcium and vitamin D alone can help reduce the rate of bone fractures is rather limited. The fact is that a large proportion of individuals in northern latitudes and in the industrial world spend inadequate time getting the exposure to sunlight that they need to avoid vitamin D deficiency. This is true whether they are prostate cancer patients or not. Thus, we continue to support patients on ADT getting the recommended dose of both vitamin D and calcium. However, you should not count on taking supplements alone to protect yourself from fractures. Exercises that include impact-loading of the skeleton in combination with diet are the best way we know of to keep the bones strong.

Phytonutrients

Phytonutrients ("phyto" = plant) refer to a wide range of compounds naturally found in plant foods that promote health and are associated with a lower risk of cancer. Phytonutrients are different from vitamins and minerals found in plant foods, but phytonutrients also have health benefits. Although a variety of plant foods provide phytonutrients, some of the richest sources are also the most colorful fruits and vegetables—as well as cruciferous vegetables such as broccoli, cauliflower, cabbage, and kale.

Before covering a few more items, it is worth revisiting a point made in the introduction to this chapter, which sometimes gets missed in discussions of phytonutrients and cancer. Although foods rich in antioxidants may lower the risk of getting cancer, there is no convincing evidence that a diet rich in vegetables or even a vegan diet alone will cure prostate cancer. No foods rich in phytonutrients are known to cure prostate cancer and there are no foods or supplements known to be more beneficial than an overall well-balanced diet.

Polyphenols

Polyphenols are antioxidants found in many fruits and vegetables and are known to reduce the risk of getting cancer, at least in animal studies. Antioxidants protect your cells from damage that can lead to disease. The isoflavones found in soy are an example of compounds with strong antioxidant properties. Cruciferous vegetables, such as broccoli, cauliflower, cabbage, and kale, are high in antioxidants, but they are found in many other foods.

Punicalagin and Ellagic Acid

Pomegranate is a rich source of polyphenols including the antioxidant punicalagin. A second type of polyphenol, ellagic acid, can be found in the red berrylike seeds inside the pomegranate fruit. In spite of some promising early research with animals and human cells in the laboratory, however, to date research has not demonstrated clear benefits of pomegranate juice in men treated for prostate cancer. As with all juices, pomegranate juice is high in sugar and lacks fiber; thus, many of the benefits of eating whole fruits or vegetables are lost. It is best to focus on variety and choose whole fruits and vegetables more often and limit your intake of juices.

Lycopene

Lycopene is a type of polyphenol antioxidant found primarily in tomatoes. It is what makes them red. It also occurs in papaya, grapefruit, and watermelon, but not in strawberries or cherries. It should be noted that grapefruit may interact with certain medications such as those to treat high cholesterol or blood pressure, among others, so you may want to check with your pharmacist. Research into the links between lycopene and prostate cancer prevention is promising. Although not all studies agree, collectively the data suggest that lycopene intake is associated with a reduced risk of getting prostate cancer and may be somewhat protective against it being aggressive.

Tomatoes and other fruits also contain a wide range of other nutrients important to health and are recommended as part of a diet rich in plant-based foods. We do know that lycopene from natural sources is widely available, safe to eat, and can easily be incorporated into your diet. Fresh fruits and vegetables are not necessarily, though, the best way to get lycopene. Cooked tomatoes (in sauces and juices) are better than fresh ones because lycopene is fat-soluble: Your body will absorb more lycopene when it is processed with a little oil. Cooking tomatoes is also preferred, since heat releases lycopene from inside the plant cells. It is best to select low-salt, low-sugar versions of tomato juice, sauce, and paste.

The following table will help you determine the lycopene concentration in common foods. Because the specific role of lycopene in disease prevention has not been established, daily intake or dietary allowance recommendations have not been established.

Food	Measure	Lycopene Content (mg)
Vegetable juice cocktail	1 cup	23
Tomato juice	1 cup	22
Pasta sauce	½ cup	22
Watermelon	1 wedge (about 286 g)	13
Tomato soup (canned, made with milk)	1 cup	13
Stewed tomatoes	1 cup	10
Raw tomato	1 tomato (about 123 g)	3
Ketchup	1 tbsp	3
Grapefruit	½ grapefruit (about 123 g)	2

Making lifestyle changes in order to eat better, like those suggested in this chapter, can be challenging. You may have trouble convincing yourself that it is worthwhile. This is a good opportunity to use a Pros/Cons table to convince yourself that for all the effort, the benefits will outweigh the inconvenience. Involve your partner and/or your other loved ones to support you in your decision, and maybe they will make the change to eating healthy with you. Know that it gets easier with time, as your new lifestyle becomes a habit.

Activity: Pros/Cons Table

Managing the side effects of ADT often requires making substantial changes to one's lifestyle. Sometimes, even though you *want* to make a lifestyle change, you may need to persuade yourself that the change is in fact worthwhile. The Pros/Cons table can be helpful in evaluating a decision to change your eating habits. Here is an example of such a table:

	PROS	CONS
MAKING THE CHANGE: Eating at home more	• better for my health • save money • spend more time with my partner cooking in the kitchen • learn a new skill • feel a stronger sense of control in my life, and better about the healthy decision I have made	• requires effort • requires more planning • takes time
STAYING THE SAME: Continuing to eat out routinely	• easier; requires less effort • get to keep eating foods I enjoy	• I will probably gain weight • feel concerned about health risks or disappointed in myself for not changing

Now, try it out for yourself.

	PROS	CONS
MAKING THE CHANGE:		
STAYING THE SAME:		

Healthy Eating   81

Activity: Action Plan

The concept of Action Plans was introduced in more detail in Chapter 2 on page 34. Here is an example of how you might complete an Action Plan to make healthy eating choices.

Action Plan Example: Reduce Eating Out

What I plan to do:_____
_____

When I plan to do it: _____
_____

Who I might do it with:_____
_____

Where I plan to do it: _____
_____

Why my plan is important:_____
_____

What might get in the way: _____
_____

How I will address what might get in the way: _____
_____

Activity: Goal Setting and Confidence

First, identify which of your goals you are rating. In order to support your goal, it is helpful to ask yourself how confident you are that you can be successful in making this change.
    Write down your goal.

Goal: _____
   (e.g., reduce frequency of eating out)

  i) Rate how confident you feel that you will achieve your nutrition goal:
     1   2   3   4   5   6   7   8   9   10
     Not confident   Very confident
 ii) Rate how motivated you are to accomplish your nutrition goal:
     1   2   3   4   5   6   7   8   9   10
     Not motivated   Very motivated
iii) Rate how likely you are to actually carry out your nutrition goal:
     1   2   3   4   5   6   7   8   9   10
     Not likely   Very likely

Healthy Eating: Essentials

ADT has several side effects that can be reduced with a well-balanced diet and a healthy lifestyle. In addition to side effects, such as loss of muscle mass and weight gained as fat, men on ADT are also at increased risk of osteoporosis, diabetes, and cardiovascular problems. In this chapter, we outlined how eating healthy can help you manage your weight and reduce these risk factors.

> **In general, you should aim for the following:**
> 1. Eat more high-fiber foods.
> 2. Eat more fish and less red meat.
> 3. Eat less saturated and trans fats.
> 4. Limit salt and sugar intake.
> 5. Eat less processed foods.

In addition, we discuss fats, proteins, and carbohydrates, as well as outline a diet for men being treated with ADT. That diet is composed of 20% to 35% fat (no more than 10% from saturated sources), 10% to 35% protein, and 45% to 65% carbohydrates. Add foods rich in phytonutrients, such as soy and tomatoes, to your diet. Also include 1,500 to 2,000 IU of vitamin D per day alongside no more than 1,500 to 2,000 mg calcium per day from all sources, unless otherwise advised by your physician. These are important components of a healthy diet for men on ADT, in particular for bone health.

Moving Forward: Questions for Discussion

- What has been my daily caloric intake for the past 3 days?
- Did I get any soy in my diet? If so, how many different forms of soy have I eaten in the last week? If I have not been eating soy, what is one way that I could introduce it into my diet this coming week?
- What actions have I taken (or can I take) to cut back on the amount of saturated fats that I have eaten in the past 3 days?
- What are some foods that I can eat to introduce more natural sources of calcium into my diet?
- How many servings of fish have I eaten in the last week?
- Are there opportunities for me to reduce my salt or sugar intake?
- What are some ways I can become more involved in grocery shopping and meal planning so as to rely less on prepared/convenience food items and eating out?
- What are some of the lasting mental health benefits that I might begin to notice if I start eating better?

NOTES

5

EFFECTS ON PSYCHOLOGICAL WELL-BEING

A diagnosis of cancer and subsequent adjustment to the effects of cancer treatment often leaves patients and loved ones feeling stressed, which can come to the surface as changes in emotions and mood. Both patients and their partners report changes in the emotions of men starting on androgen deprivation therapy (ADT). These are often in the form of mood swings or increased emotional expression, often referred to as *emotional lability*. It is perfectly normal for you to experience abrupt mood changes, depression, anxiety, and grief while on ADT. It is important for you to be aware of this and to be open to discussing changes in emotional responses or sensitivity that might occur.

Emotional lability can create challenges for relationships. If the patient thinks that his new and heightened emotions are wrong and must be hidden or denied, his desire to draw on social support from others can be compromised. Patients may also experience depression, anxiety, and grief that can be difficult to adjust to. We have found in our research though that if men are experiencing emotional changes related to ADT, whether they are distressing to him or not, a couple can maintain a good cosupportive relationship as long as he and his partner are aware of those changes.

Emotional changes can be quite variable. Some men may become angry, bitter, and/or pessimistic while on ADT. Others may become more sentimental and openly tearful. Often, partners or close friends see the changes before the patient himself notices.

ADT may also impact a patient's **cognitive function**, which refers to conscious thinking processes such as attention, concentration, and memory. The research examining the nature of these changes during ADT is inconsistent. It is hard to know if changes in cognitive function are natural responses to aging or are brought on by stress, anxiety, depression, and/or fatigue. However, we do know that ADT can be associated with cognitive changes above and beyond just aging. We believe that you should be aware that ADT *might* affect cognitive function, though we do not know how common such changes in cognitive function are with ADT. If you do notice cognitive changes, such as memory loss, it is also unknown how long those changes may last.

Emotional Distress

When your prostate-specific antigen (PSA) rises after completion of primary treatments, such as prostatectomy or radiotherapy, having to start or resume ADT can be associated with significant distress for both you and your loved ones. At this point, we know that the previous, potentially curative, treatments are no longer an option. Some despair is understandable in this situation. These feelings should be balanced against the reality that ADT can help control your cancer for many years, if not decades, to come.

A common stressor for prostate cancer patients centers on having blood drawn for a PSA test and then needing to wait for the results. Patients on ADT are required to have regular PSA tests, and that alone can contribute significantly to the emotional burden of being on ADT.

You are also likely to experience additional stress at various points in the course of your treatment. These reactions are realistic in response to a difficult situation. However, if you find that you are significantly distressed, you should consider additional treatment for depression and/or anxiety, for example, seeing a professional counselor.

> **We cannot tell you how you will react to emotional changes that may come with ADT, but we can say that your willingness to talk about such changes can help bring you closer to your loved ones. Others will appreciate you sharing your feelings with them.**
>
> **At the other extreme, if you feel that you need to deny or hide such changes from your loved ones, it could make things confusing and frustrating for both of you. Partners often report that patient withdrawal is the hardest thing for them to deal with.**

Emotional Expression

Spontaneous tearfulness is commonly reported by ADT patients, perhaps because it is a noticeable sign of emotional change. In mainstream culture, men or women may feel that it is "unmanly" for a man to shed tears. In reality, there are various reasons why anyone might cry (e.g., physical discomfort, sadness, joy). If you as a patient start to find yourself crying about something that you might never have cried about before, it can be helpful to determine what caused that moment of tearfulness.

One patient on ADT told us that he never teared up because of pain or self-pity; rather, he became tearful in response to news stories and TV advertisements that focused on the triumphs and tribulations of humankind. This patient interpreted his occasional spontaneous tearfulness as a demonstration of heightened empathy for others, and subsequently took personal pride in his newly acquired sensitivity. He now shares tissues with his partner during sentimental movies, and they both feel closer because of his new ability to both show and share emotional responsiveness.

Another patient saw any tendency for tearfulness as a sign of lost masculine strength. He became embarrassed when his family saw him become tearful, and then got angry with himself for being seen as emotional. He withdrew from his family and would not talk about what happened or how he felt, which pained those who cared about him.

A third patient reported increased expression of anger. This patient told us that he had always been calm and slow to respond when angry. Now he acknowledged that he was shouting and slamming doors. His family had a difficult time figuring out what had changed. Such changes can be confusing for patients, partners, family members, and close friends who have not anticipated the emotional lability that ADT can bring on.

Activity: Self-Assessment—Screening for Emotional Distress

Many patients and their loved ones experience significant emotional distress when dealing with cancer treatments and ADT. If you are interested in doing a self-assessment, the following questionnaires will give you an idea of how you are doing. Regardless of whether or not you or your loved ones choose to fill out these questionnaires, you may still find it valuable to continue reading the rest of the chapter.

The following questionnaire, known as the Patient Health Questionnaire (PHQ-9), assesses different aspects of one's mood. Indicate your response using the categories on the right and circle the number that best represents your experience.

How often have you experienced the following problems in the past 2 weeks?

	Not at All	Several Days	More Than Half the Days	Nearly Every Day
1. Little interest or pleasure in doing things	0	1	2	3
2. Feeling down, depressed, or hopeless	0	1	2	3
3. Trouble falling asleep or staying asleep, or sleeping too much	0	1	2	3
4. Feeling tired or having little energy	0	1	2	3
5. Poor appetite or overeating	0	1	2	3
6. Feeling bad about yourself, or that you are a failure, or that you have let yourself or your family down	0	1	2	3
7. Trouble concentrating on things such as reading the newspaper or watching television	0	1	2	3
8. Moving or speaking so slowly that other people could have noticed. Or the opposite—being so fidgety or restless that you have been moving around a lot more than usual	0	1	2	3
9. Thoughts that you would be better off dead or of hurting yourself in some way	0	1	2	3
Column Totals:		____ +	____ +	____
Add Column Totals Together:		____		

Scoring Instructions:

- Scores below 5 indicate no concern.
- Scores between 5 and 14 indicate some mild symptoms of difficulty with mood. You may be able to address these by seeking support from family and friends, beginning to work through a self-help book (see the Resources section on page 173 for suggestions), or making efforts to engage in more rewarding and pleasurable activities in your life.
- Scores of 15 or higher indicate symptoms of depression and likely warrant seeking help from a professional counselor and/or physician.

The following questionnaire known as the Generalized Anxiety Disorder 7-Item Scale (GAD-7) also assesses symptoms of distress. Using the categories on the right, indicate the most applicable answer for each item.

How often have you experienced the following problems in the past 2 weeks?

	Not at All	Several Days	More Than Half the Days	Nearly Every Day
1. Feeling nervous, anxious, or on edge	0	1	2	3
2. Not being able to stop or control worrying	0	1	2	3
3. Worrying too much about different things	0	1	2	3
4. Trouble relaxing	0	1	2	3
5. Being so restless that it is hard to sit still	0	1	2	3
6. Becoming easily annoyed or irritable	0	1	2	3
7. Feeling afraid, as if something awful might happen	0	1	2	3
Column Totals:		____ +	____ +	____
Add Totals Together:		____		

Scoring Instructions:

- Scores below 5 indicate no concern.
- Scores between 5 and 10 indicate some mild symptoms of difficulty with stress. You may be able to address these by seeking support from family and friends, beginning to work through a self-help book (see the Resources section on page 173 for suggestions), or practicing the relaxation exercises on pages 91–94.
- Scores over 10 indicate symptoms of anxiety and warrant seeking help from a professional counselor and/or physician.

Depression

Increasingly, the medical literature has reported an association of ADT with an increased risk of depression, and the risk increases the longer one is on ADT. It is clear that not all men become depressed on ADT and the various studies provide different estimates of how common it is. However, one massive study that combined the results of 18 previous studies totaling data from over 168,000 men reported a 41% increase in the risk of depression. That is common enough that it is important to discuss with your physician if you are feeling depressed or have a low mood. There are interventions that can be helpful, including increased physical activity, psychological counseling, and pharmaceutical treatments.

Depression in men on ADT rarely appears as a single problem. More often, fatigue, insomnia, and depression form a triad of interrelated symptoms. Because one or more of these complications is frequently a side effect of treatment, it can be difficult to distinguish the primary cause(s) from subsequent effect(s). Depression, when it occurs, may be an indirect, but entirely realistic, emotional reaction to the situation that ADT patients find themselves in; that is, it may be a response to a cancer diagnosis and the many changes that it can bring to the lives of all those that it touches.

Some studies, however, suggest that low testosterone in men, even if they are not cancer patients, is associated with greater feelings of sadness and low mood. New research also suggests that insulin resistance (diabetes) and a tendency toward depression may be linked. This is another reason why exercise, which helps regulate blood sugar, is so important for the physical and psychological well-being of men on ADT.

Note that rates of depression in the *partners* of cancer patients are often as high as the rates in patients. In fact, one study with prostate cancer couples showed that depression in the partners of patients on ADT was higher than for the patients themselves. Partners may feel depressed for various reasons related to the patient's cancer diagnosis, such as fear of the disease progressing, financial burden associated with treatments, or the intimate and relationship changes due to ADT. Therefore, it *is* important for partners to seek treatment as well, if they feel depressed.

Overall, both patients and partners should be concerned about changes in vitality and spirit. Watch for any of these signs of depression in yourself. You can also watch for these changes in your loved ones:

- Feeling too tired and gloomy to exercise.
- Feeling sadness that does not seem to dissipate.
- Becoming withdrawn and noncommunicative.
- Losing interest in a range of personal activities that were previously enjoyable.
- Feeling worthless, guilty, and hopeless.
- Having diminished ability to concentrate or make decisions.
- Increased alcohol consumption.

Anxiety

Psychologists have characterized depression as a state of mind provoked by excessive, repetitive thoughts and concerns about the *past*. This contrasts with what is considered to provoke anxiety; that is, excessive, repetitive thoughts and concerns about the *future*. Depression and anxiety often coexist, and may be expressed in similar ways. This can make it particularly hard to decipher the causes for a change in mood.

One recent study reported that ADT raises the risk of not just depression, but also anxiety in men. Similar to depression, the risk of anxiety increased with longer duration ADT. However, another study found that anxiety levels that were high at the start of ADT actually came down after 6 months. The differences between the studies may reflect differences in the contexts for the patients starting on ADT in the first place. If patients are anxious because of a rising PSA and ADT brings their PSA down, that alone could reduce anxiety.

If you feel anxious about starting ADT, be aware of the increase in stress in your life associated with the transition to ADT, and remain determined to find time to rest and relax. Some of the best treatments for anxiety and depression include eating healthy, exercising, having someone to talk to, medication, and/or counseling. Watch for any of these signs of anxiety in yourself and your loved ones:

- Worrying excessively about the future for an extended period of time.
- Fear of "going crazy" or losing control.
- Feeling "on edge" or that you just cannot relax.
- Having difficulty in sleeping.
- Feeling that your mind is racing.

To live well on ADT, it is important to maintain an active lifestyle and nurture genuine communication with your loved ones. Depression and anxiety can hinder both. The most effective treatment for depression and anxiety involves medication paired with psychotherapy or counseling. Exercise and healthy eating are also effective.

Talk to your doctor, psychologist, or counselor if you are suffering. Timely treatment can set you free to enjoy life again.

Activity: Progressive Muscle Relaxation

This exercise is to help you learn how to relax your body and mind. Developed by Edmund Jacobsen in the 1920s, *progressive muscle relaxation* is a well-known exercise in which a person tenses and then relaxes the various muscle groups in the body. If you have any pain or discomfort, move on to another muscle group. It may be helpful if, throughout this exercise, you visualize the muscles tensing and then a wave of relaxation flowing over you as you release the tension. Remember to breathe throughout the exercise; do not hold your breath.

Physical tension in the body occurs when we are anxious or stressed. We are often not aware of the tension we hold in our head, jaw, neck, and shoulders until someone brings it to our attention; we do not think to relax these muscle groups. This exercise can be practiced whether you are sitting in a chair or lying down. Make sure to choose a comfortable position. After you have read these instructions, you may choose to practice with your eyes closed, if you are comfortable doing so.

You may not want to practice this exercise if you are prone to muscle spasms, or if you have pain from an existing injury.

1. Begin by creating a tight fist with your hands. Hold your arms out straight in front of you and hold this tension. Take note of what the tightness in your muscles feels like. Hold for at least 10 seconds. As you breathe out, relax your fists and let go of any tension you were holding. If you are sitting, allow your arms to fall to your sides and feel the muscles go limp. It is important to deliberately focus on the difference between the tension and relaxation in your muscles. Rest for 20 to 30 seconds.
2. Now move your attention to your feet. Scrunch up your toes into a ball. Then, tense up your ankles, pointing your toes toward your nose. Feel the stretch in the muscles of your calves as you do this. Hold for 10 seconds. Then, while exhaling, release the tension and rest for 20 to 30 seconds.
3. Move your attention up to your thighs and buttocks. Tighten up these muscles so that your body weight is lifted off the surface you are sitting or lying on. Squeeze your thighs together and hold for 10 seconds. Now exhale and feel the release of the tension. Rest for 20 to 30 seconds.
4. Move your attention now to your abdomen. Imagine bringing your belly button closer to your spine and straighten your body. Hold this posture for 10 seconds. Then exhale, releasing the muscle tension and letting all the muscles of your belly (body wall) become loose; feel the tension disappear. Rest here for 20 to 30 seconds.
5. Next, move to your shoulders. Scrunch them up as close to your ears as you can and squeeze your upper arms against your ribcage. Hold for 10 seconds. Exhale, releasing the tension and letting your arms relax away from your body. If you are sitting, let your shoulders fall. Rest for 20 to 30 seconds.
6. Now squeeze the muscles in your face. Scrunch up your forehead, eyebrows, eyes, and lips. Close your mouth and gently bite down. Hold for 10 seconds. As you exhale, release the tension and relax for 20 to 30 seconds.

Take a quick mental scan of your body, noting any areas where you are still holding or feeling any tension. Often, as we adjust to relax one area of our body, we begin to tense another area without being aware that we are doing so. Repeat any of the previous steps to ensure that you have let go of all of the tension in that muscle group. Try to perform this progressive muscle relaxation once or twice daily.

Like other things in life, practicing this exercise will improve your skill with it over time. When you begin, it may take you 20 minutes to complete the exercise and even then you may not become fully relaxed. With consistent practice, though, you will find that it takes you only a few minutes to fully relax. An alternative relaxation exercise is the abdominal breathing technique detailed on pages 20 to 21 as a treatment for hot flashes. Introducing relaxation exercises or deep breathing into your daily routine may help you to manage overall chronic stress or anxiety.

Activity: Mindfulness Meditation

One strategy to cope with increased stress is to start a mindfulness meditation practice. Research has demonstrated that mindfulness can help in the treatment of depression, anxiety, insomnia, and chronic pain. Mindful awareness, as with any skill, is developed with practice. We spend much of our lives functioning on "auto-pilot" or engaging in "multi-tasking," trying to spread our attention across many different activities at once, without being truly aware of what we are doing in the moment. Mindful awareness exercises help us to develop the ability to focus on physical sensations in the body and teach us how to deal with thoughts and emotions that interrupt our physical experience. Through mindful awareness we turn our attention toward sensations of touch, sight, sound, and so on. Rather than following distractions in thoughts, getting hung up on judgments, or focusing on feelings about your experience (or even thoughts about other topics entirely), individuals can train themselves to bring their attention fully to the physical sensations they are experiencing at the moment.

Instructions

This exercise is designed to heighten awareness of your moment-by-moment experience and to become more in touch with the present. If your mind wanders during this exercise, this is fine; just bring your attention back to the activity at hand. If practicing this activity on your own, make sure you are seated comfortably, with your back against your chair and your feet placed on the ground. Or you can try this exercise lying down. Close your eyes if you feel more comfortable doing so.

1. Begin by paying attention to your breath. Do not try to change it in any way; just start to bring awareness to your breathing. Pay attention to how your chest expands when you breathe in and how it falls as you breathe out. Notice the sensation of the air as it passes into and out of your nostrils each time you inhale and exhale. If that is uncomfortable for you, try breathing in through your nose and out through your mouth.

2. Begin to check in with your five senses. What do you hear? Can you label what those noises or distractions are? Can you taste or smell anything? If you do smell something, have you judged it to be positive or negative?
3. Begin to tune into your bodily sensations. Can you feel anything going on in your body? Can you feel your pulse? Is your stomach grumbling? Do you have an itch? Acknowledge these sensations.
4. Begin to become aware of your body's position in the chair or on the bed. Notice your legs and feet. Notice where your feet/legs contact the ground or bed. Take note of your thighs and buttocks, or whatever part of your body rests on the surface beneath you. Notice how the surface holds the weight of your body.
5. Shift your attention to your hands. Are your hands resting on an armrest? Are they on your lap? Are they resting beside your body? What do they feel? Can your hands feel a certain texture? Is it rough or smooth? Soft or firm? Are they warm or cold?
6. Do you have any urges to move or change position to become more comfortable? If so, scratch an itch or adjust your posture accordingly. However, be conscious of your choice to do this rather than just responding to the body in an automatic fashion. Be intentional in your motions and pay attention to the sensations of movement as you move your body.
7. When you feel ready, bring your attention back to the room and to your environment. Notice how refreshed and peaceful you feel, ready to carry on with the day.

Further Developing Your Mindfulness Practice

We recommend that patients and family distressed about cancer look into a short course on mindful meditation. Increasingly, hospitals that treat cancer patients and other healthcare centers are offering such courses. There are also many video resources that can be found online and used to help you develop your mindfulness meditation practice—the script we have provided is only one option. See additional resources at the end of this book.

Fatigue

You should not confuse the bodily feeling of muscle fatigue that you get at the end of a strenuous exercise session with the fatigue that comes from not exercising. Pushing your body by exercising increases blood flow to the muscles you are working, as well as to the brain. Right after exercising in this way, your body may feel tired, but you will sleep better and your brain will feel more alert in the following days. We can also differentiate between mental and physical fatigue, though both are likely to co-occur. Mental fatigue is often associated with cognitive symptoms such as poor concentration and/or forgetfulness or emotional exhaustion, which can show up as feelings of discouragement, cynicism, or detachment.

Grief

Cancer and cancer treatments bring with them many changes, including changes interpreted as losses. With ADT, changes that affect how a man feels in terms of his vitality and sexuality may surface. For some men these changes are minor, but for many they are very significant. Many men may find it difficult to accept transitions or losses brought on by ADT that affect their core identity and sense of self. Similarly, partners of patients may also experience grief due to the changes they observe in the patient. These may arise because of changes in how the patient interacts with them.

It is okay to grieve losses. In fact, much has been written in the cancer literature about how important grieving is to the process of recovering from loss. Grieving is therapeutic.

Among the changes associated with ADT, there are those linked with a man's body image, as well as a man's sense of physical strength and masculinity. ADT can change how a man's body feels, and how he feels about his body. These changes can negatively impact a patient's mood, attitude, and thoughts; and how a man thinks and feels about both himself and his partner. How easily you, either as a patient or as a loved one, adapt to these changes can be influenced by how willing you are to acknowledge and accept the changes in the first place.

Grieving losses from ADT can be difficult because the changes may be more internal and emotional, and hard to articulate to others or even to oneself. Patients on ADT typically know they have changed, but for many it is not easy to describe exactly how they are experiencing those changes.

After the effects of ADT take shape, you may find it helpful to make a list of the things you consider lost or reduced due to ADT. Some examples may be physical strength, loss of spontaneous sex, decreased erectile function, loss of libido, and changes to your body form and physical appearance.

> **People grieve in different ways—some may cry about a specific loss, while others may choose a designated time to remember and celebrate the ways things were. Other individuals may reframe loss so they see it as a benefit. Discuss what each loss or change means to both you and your loved ones. Then you can make the decision to move ahead with life together, despite those changes.**

One of the obstacles to living comfortably with change is an all-too-common effort to try to reestablish or reaffirm life as it was before ADT. Too often this requires pretending that life has not changed. On the surface this may work for

> **The more that patients use denial to deal with the changes that ADT brings to their lives, the less they can grieve. This makes it that much more difficult for them to adapt to the changes they are experiencing and to recover from their losses.**

the patient, but for partners and loved ones a patient's silence and reluctance to acknowledge change can make the grieving process all that more difficult.

Men often engage in a code of silence. Because men rarely talk with others about aspects of their lives that make them feel less manly, men on ADT may feel culturally trapped into pretending that their lives have not changed. The more that men are reluctant to reveal how they feel after going on ADT, the more other patients assume that being silent is the right thing—the "manly" thing—to do. This leads to a vicious cycle, where masculine culture can make it particularly difficult for patients to acknowledge change and loss during ADT. This traps men into denying change and hiding how they really feel.

> **Adapting well to ADT often involves sharing your grief with someone. If you have a partner, it means that both of you are willing to share with and support each other in whatever grief you each may experience along the way. Although this can be painful emotionally, the end product is often a couple that is closer and more supportive of each other than ever before.**
>
> **If you share your concerns with a loved one, you may find that your relationships are stronger, not weaker, after ADT. This may allow you to better accept the changes and losses you experience as a result of ADT.**

Grief is interlinked with emotional expression. If men feel that it is unmanly to display emotion, yet inside they feel a loss, they may hold their grief inside. Typically, partners know that the patients are troubled by the changes in their lives brought on by their cancer treatment. But if the patients themselves are reluctant to talk about how they are experiencing these changes, partners may feel that the best they can do is to join their men in pretending that little has changed. Ultimately, in this situation, the couple moves farther apart rather than closer together. It is at times like this when couples counseling can be beneficial.

Cognition

There are more than a dozen research studies that have explored whether ADT with luteinizing hormone-releasing hormone (LHRH) agonist drugs are linked to cognitive problems (for example, memory function). Those studies have mixed results. One study found no evidence of cognitive effects and another even suggested some improvement, but it was a small study. The length of the studies is also a factor. The studies tended to show little or no changes for the first 6 months, but more significant changes when the data were collected at 12 months after starting on ADT. Therefore, the duration of ADT may influence the extent of cognitive problems. Taking all these things into consideration, there seems to be evidence that patients on ADT may experience some declines in cognitive processes. Unfortunately, the various researchers have measured cognitive effects in different ways, leading to a confusing picture about how ADT affects men's thought processes and memory. In an effort to clarify the situation, researchers recently compiled all the studies into one large analysis (called a "**meta-analysis**"), which allows researchers to produce more rigorous conclusions. The meta-analysis suggested that there can indeed be cognitive effects from the long-term use of LHRH agonist drugs, but the effects are subtle and vary greatly from patient to patient. The strongest evidence links the long-term use of ADT with changes in visual-spatial processing. Studies on nonprostate cancer patients are consistent with that and have found some correlation between testosterone levels and navigational skill.

In everyday life, changes in visual-spatial processing can manifest themselves as problems such as not remembering where you left your car keys, important papers, or stuff in the refrigerator. Visual-spatial processing can also extend to skills such as assembling puzzles that require good spatial skills or even following a map. The ability to remember the placement of objects—be they the keys to the car or the car in a large parking lot—may be influenced by ADT. However, some of the presumed cognitive impairment with ADT can be attributed to aging, stress, and illness in general.

Despite the fact that the cognitive effects of ADT are not well defined, there are ways that may help improve or maintain cognitive function, should you experience such problems. The following suggestions are potentially preventative and are likely to be most effective if started early before cognitive changes affect one's daily life.

- *Maintain an active lifestyle*. Exercise improves blood flow to the brain, which helps your brain to work more efficiently, improving cognitive abilities such as memory, attention, and concentration.
- *Keep your brain active*. Do activities that make your brain work, including reading and conversing with others. Puzzles and games (e.g., sudoku, crossword puzzles, bridge, scrabble) can help you maintain spatial and verbal skills. A variety of games that challenge different parts of your brain (e.g., mathematical ability, memory, logic puzzles, word games) may be best.
- *Be practical*. For example, it helps to have a standard place to keep your car keys. Keep a notebook and pen or pencil by the telephone to write down messages. Get rid of clutter on your desk to help you find things more easily.
- *Focus by avoiding multitasking*. If you have something important to write or to read (like this book!), give it your full attention without TV, radio, or other distracting noises in the background.
- *Write important things down*. For example, write your appointments on a calendar that you keep clearly visible, or write them down in an agenda. When you have something important to note, write it as soon as possible; otherwise, you may forget about it when you get distracted by other things.

- *Medications.* There are medications that are being developed to help slow the mental decline that we all experience with aging. Some drugs are already marketed to treat mild dementia, but there have not been well-designed studies of these agents to know if they are truly effective and also safe for men on ADT. So far, one small, short-term study has suggested that estradiol can help slow memory decline from ADT.

Finally, there is some evidence that hearing loss can exacerbate cognitive decline. When one cannot hear conversations he or she may be inclined to withdraw from social situations and become isolated. If you feel like you are having problems hearing, we encourage you to get your hearing checked. Although this has not been explicitly assessed for men on ADT, the argument has been made that hearing aids can improve cognitive functioning.

Activity: Pros/Cons Table

If you have been reading through this book chapter by chapter, you are familiar with the value of the Pros/Cons table by now. This exercise can be applied to any decision in your life. The following is an example of the Pros/Cons table related to addressing emotional concerns.

	PROS	CONS
MAKING THE CHANGE: Seeing a counselor	• They might have ideas about how to help me deal with stress • They might be able to assure me that I am doing just fine and then I do not have to worry • They might be able to provide additional support for my partner • My partner might be relieved that I am getting support	• It could be embarrassing to ask for help • Have to take time out of my schedule for appointments • There may be an additional cost
DO NOT CHANGE: Continue without seeing a counselor	• I do not have to face the reality that maybe I need some extra support • I do not have to feel embarrassed	• I might continue to struggle • I feel overwhelmed and unsupported • My partner feels overwhelmed trying to support me

Now, try it out for yourself.

	PROS	CONS
MAKING THE CHANGE:		
STAYING THE SAME:		

Activity: Action Plan

Again you are reminded that it is best to start small with something very manageable (e.g., walking regularly) before you take on larger scale goals (e.g., running a 10-km race). Post your completed form somewhere where you will see it every day, like next to your bathroom mirror, to remind yourself of your commitment to this goal.

Action Plan Example: Work on Stress Management

What I plan to do: use the progressive muscle relaxation exercise regularly

When I plan to do it: every day at lunch break for 10 minutes

Who I might do it with: by myself

Where I plan to do it: at my desk, with the door closed, after I have eaten my lunch

Why my plan is important: to improve my ability to manage chronic stress and to build my relaxation skills

What might get in the way: people might think I am weird, or wonder what I am doing

How I will address what might get in the way: I will close my office door

Following is a blank copy that you can fill out. An additional copy is located in the Appendix on page 162. It helps to be as specific as possible when you are making your Action Plan.

Action Plan:

What I plan to do: _____

_____

When I plan to do it: _____

_____

Who I might do it with: _____

_____

Where I plan to do it: _____

_____

Why my plan is important: _____

_____

What might get in the way: _____

_____

How I will address what might get in the way: _____

_____

Activity: Goal Setting and Confidence

In order to support your goal, take a moment to rate the following factors associated with your goal. First, write down your goal (this might be what you have written in your Action Plan):

Goal _____

i) Rate how confident you feel that you will achieve your goal:
    1   2   3   4   5   6   7   8   9   10
    Not confident   Very confident

ii) Rate how motivated you are to accomplish your goal:
    1   2   3   4   5   6   7   8   9   10
    Not motivated   Very motivated

iii) Rate how likely you are to actually carry out your goal:
    1   2   3   4   5   6   7   8   9   10
    Not likely   Very likely

If any of your answers *are less than five*:

- Consider either enlisting the help of a friend to hold you accountable or implementing a reward system to help motivate you (see pages 57 to 58 for additional information on motivation, lapses, relapses, rewards, and support).
- Consider revising your goal—Is it too ambitious a goal to start with? Can you start with a more modest goal and work your way up to a more significant lifestyle change?
- Remind yourself—What are the reasons? Why do you want to make this change? What potential benefits may you notice? List these on a piece of paper or smartphone and refer back to them when you are feeling particularly unmotivated.
- Consider completing the previous Pros/Cons table to help you identify your motivations (pros) for making this change, but also some of the barriers (cons) that might be getting in the way of making the change.

Effects on Psychological Well-Being: Essentials

Some patients report that they experience no changes in their mood, emotions, or thought process while on ADT. Others notice significant changes that make them uncomfortable. In some cases, the patients may not notice changes in their mood or thought processes, but their loved ones and others close to them may be the first to notice the psychological changes. We encourage you to be aware of the possibility of change, and should changes occur, take simple steps to address and accommodate them.

Some of the psychological changes that can occur with ADT, such as depression or anxiety, can be helped by exercise, medication, and counseling. If changes in memory occur, they can often be compensated for by small changes in lifestyle and working habits. Planning can be a very important factor in adapting successfully to change. Remember to talk to your healthcare team if these problems arise so that they can be addressed properly.

Emotional changes (particularly increased tearfulness), although common, are not necessarily negative. They can even be seen as enriching your life if you accept them as positive signs of your sensitivity to others, and not as a loss of masculine detachment and reserve.

Changes in mood, emotions, or cognition are often very subtle and may be noticed by a partner or loved one before they are noticed or acknowledged by a patient. Not talking about these changes when they are obvious to others can hurt relationships. They are not uniformly bad, and they do not need to be hidden. Talking about any changes is very important for adapting to them.

Moving Forward: Questions for Discussion

Emotional Changes

- How will I acknowledge and communicate with my loved ones about any changes in my mood and emotions that I experience while on ADT?
- How do I feel about increased emotional expression?
- What will I do if I become depressed or experience anxiety?
- How much will I share with my loved ones if I am depressed or experiencing anxiety?
- What will I do if my loved ones become depressed or experience anxiety?
- What things have I lost since having cancer and starting ADT?
- What can I do to help grieve something that I have lost?

Cognitive Changes

- How do I feel about cognitive changes, for example, increased forgetfulness?
- What can I incorporate into my life to prevent or reduce the impact of cognitive changes?
- What changes can I make around the house or office to help me if cognitive changes occur?
- How will I explain this effect of ADT to my friends and family if they notice a change?

NOTES:

6

EFFECTS ON INTIMATE RELATIONSHIPS AND SEXUALITY

This chapter is relevant to both straight and gay men who are either partnered or single, whether or not they had already stopped having partnered sex prior to the start of androgen deprivation therapy (ADT). We have found that a loss of libido changes most men's relationships—even for those who were not previously sexually active.

This chapter also includes a section specifically on dating (see pages 108–109). Whether you have a regular partner now or not, you may find this section relevant.

Whether you participate in partnered sexual activities or not you will likely notice changes to your sexuality when you are on ADT.

One partner shared with us: "I was very afraid of living together like siblings. It feels like you're going to move into this platonic sort of relationship where there's none of that wonderful thing you had as a married couple."

ADT Lowers Libido

Approximately 90% of men on ADT experience a reduced libido (desire for or interest in sex). A reduction in libido typically leads to decreased frequency or, in some cases, a complete cessation of sexual activity. Reduced libido can also lead to fewer displays of physical affection within a partnership. Therefore, ADT may thus affect both patients and their sexual partners when the patients' sexual desire diminishes.

How the Loss of Libido Affects Couples

Couples respond to the loss of libido from ADT in many different ways:

- Some couples may not be sexually active at the time of treatment and may notice little change.
- Some couples readily accept the loss of sex in exchange for a potentially longer life.
- Some couples may stop having sex and find that they experience sorrow and mourn the loss of their sex life.
- With the loss of sexual intimacy, some couples stop being physically affectionate and this can contribute to a sense of disconnection between partners.
- Some couples redefine their sexual activity and find new meaning in those activities that they are still able to do.

One patient said that he likes that he can cuddle up with his partner and enjoy closeness without the "carry-on of the last 30 years trying to plan how ... to get my partner to have sex."

As a patient on ADT, you may feel that you have lost your zest for life. You may no longer find delight in flirting because it does not feel genuine. If you have a regular partner, she or he may feel grief over the loss of the glances and touches that you used to share. This may lead your partner to feel less appreciated, attractive, or desired. Changes in libido and/or sexual functioning can make it difficult to maintain physical and nonphysical intimacy, both of which are important for maintaining a feeling of closeness.

Here, we explore ways that patients and their partners can remain close—or perhaps become even closer—despite the impact of ADT on libido. We present a range of possibilities that require couples to remain open to discussing what a changed libido might mean to them. A prerequisite to maintaining intimacy in the face of reduced libido is communication.

Staying Close in Nonsexual Ways

Intimacy is the feeling of closeness and connection you have with a partner. Intimacy comes from sharing something with someone that you share with no one else. This includes both physical (sexual and nonsexual) and nonphysical contact. Although ADT may reduce sexual intimacy, partners can still feel very close and enjoy nonsexual and nonphysical intimacy. For most couples, intimacy is an important part of their relationship, but building intimacy does not necessarily require participating in sexual activities.

Nonphysical intimacy can increase after ADT for many reasons. For example, a cancer diagnosis itself may remind people how precious their relationships are, and a stronger mutual appreciation (one that is not driven solely by sexual desire) can develop or be strengthened. As another example, a couple may find new activities that they can do together such as exercising together or trying out new recipes. Though not explicitly sexual, these shared activities can build intimacy.

At the same time, we recognize that mismatched libidos could have been a source of tension in some partnerships prior to ADT. For example, when a man on ADT who previously had a higher sex drive now has a libido that matches his partner, this can ease tension if both partners are accepting of the change.

When ADT reduces a patient's desire for sexual intimacy and his ability to have erections, many established couples stop engaging in penetrative sexual activities. Refraining from sex is not necessarily in itself problematic. What can lead to problems is when couples in this situation become overall less physically affectionate toward each other. This can result in both partners longing for the comfort that physical affection brings, whether through cuddling, hugs, kisses, or even sexual touch and orgasm. At the same time, partners or patients may be holding back because they fear that expressing physical affection may cause anxiety, pressure, or expectations of a sexual nature. For example, the patient may think: "I don't want to be too physically affectionate because I don't want to start something sexual that I can't finish"; his partner may think: "I don't want to cuddle up to him because he'll assume it means I want sexual activity or intercourse and that will just make him feel worse."

Try discussing what you each consider to be physical affection that leads to sexual intercourse or other sexual activities, compared to physical affection that can simply be interpreted as being close and enjoying each other's warmth. You may decide that holding hands, hugging, cuddling, or kissing are physically intimate activities you can enjoy without either of you feeling obligated to move toward further sexual activity. If you communicate beforehand, and you each know which activities mean closeness without committing to sex, and which activities mean you have an interest in sex, you can reduce anxiety and false expectations. This can help you continue to enjoy each other's company and stay affectionate.

> **One man told us that without sexual urges reminding him of the importance of showing affection to his partner he seldom thought of it.**
>
> **His solution was to wear a prostate cancer bracelet on his wrist. Whenever he felt it, he either made a point of communicating something that he appreciated about his partner or touched his partner affectionately.**

The key is to communicate about your expectations and know that you can be physically affectionate without that affection needing to lead to sexual activity.

You may experience a whole range of emotions when it comes to how your sexuality has been affected by ADT. You may feel anxious about being intimate with your partner, in sexual or nonsexual ways, because your sex drive and ability to perform have been affected. You may be self-conscious about how your body or your genitals look after ADT treatment. You may be angry that you do not have the sex drive you had before going on ADT, and may feel ashamed or see yourself as less manly because of your reduced sex drive or erectile dysfunction (ED).

If you feel any of these things, it can help to acknowledge your feelings and openly discuss them with your partner. Sharing your concerns can help to build relational intimacy and also help you to cope with negative feelings.

Making Time for Intimacy

One suggestion for adapting sexually to the impact of ADT on intimacy is to choose one evening a week as a "date night." This way, you do not have to rely on your bodies reminding you to share physical intimacy, even if that intimacy is not sexual. It may help you to realize that when we are not hungry for food, looking at the clock reminds us to eat so we do not ignore our nutritional needs. When we are not hungry for sex, looking at the calendar reminds us to feed each other's need for physical and emotional intimacy, whether sexual or not. If you often feel tired in the evening, consider moving your lovemaking to the morning, when you may feel more refreshed.

> One couple told us about their sexual encounters: "We have positive experiences. I think it maintains a closeness if nothing else. Our sexual relationship is different now, but the fact that we want to give pleasure to each other is good, even if it doesn't happen very often."

Here are just a few ideas about how to "sensualize the setting":

- Put on some favorite music and dance together.
- Take a bubble bath together.
- Massage each other.
- Spend time holding each other.
- Enjoy long kisses.
- Spend time touching each other sensually.

Know that the purpose of these activities is to strengthen your physical connection—they may not, and need not, lead to more explicit sexual activities.

Dating

While we believe that single men can lead fulfilling and happy lives, we have met many single men on ADT who would like to date, but may be hesitant about starting a new relationship. Sometimes this is because they do not know where to begin telling a new partner about their cancer diagnosis or the fact that they are on ADT. They may also have fears about how to disclose sexual problems and how a new partner might react to that information. Sometimes men on ADT prematurely and unjustifiably conclude that no one would want to be in a relationship with them. There are ways to overcome these, though. Here are a few tips for single men who might be interested in dating, or seeking out new relationships.

Being Open and Honest The first step is to prepare yourself to speak openly and honestly about your medical history, which may include discussing both your cancer diagnosis and various treatments. You do not have to have a detailed script memorized about the topic. In fact, you can choose how much or how little detail you would like to share with anyone when you are first getting to know that person. However, if this is going to develop into a meaningful and lasting relationship, at some point you will need to be willing to talk about your situation.

To start with, you should be comfortable at least admitting that you have been diagnosed with prostate cancer and that you have been treated for it. It might be helpful to think ahead about how you might answer questions that a potential partner might have, such as

"How has cancer and treatment affected you?"
"What is your prognosis?"
"How are you doing now?"
"Have you noticed sexual changes?" [Reading the rest of this chapter might help you figure out how to answer questions relating to your sexual function.]

You might even try rehearsing what you might say with a trusted friend or family member. You may never get asked these questions, nor are you expected to be upbeat and endlessly positive when answering them. You should find though, in the long run, that living with ADT is easier when you can articulate to yourself and others what life is like while on ADT.

Many men wait too long to disclose their experience with prostate cancer, often because they fear rejection from a potential new partner. If this is your fear, we encourage you to consider that good, healthy relationships are based on openness and honesty. That is why we strongly encourage men to be completely honest. Potential partners most assuredly are more interested in a partner who is open and honest than one who appears to be secretive or is not open to talking about his medical history. In fact, many men have told us that when they do confide in a potential partner about their situation, the partner often reports feeling trusted and valued, and in turn becomes more comfortable with their developing relationship.

You also do not have to tell a new or potential partner everything about your cancer experience immediately. For example, when introducing yourselves over, say, a first dinner date or when writing an online dating profile, it is not required that you disclose having ED from your cancer treatment, but it is important that you do not wait too long before telling a new partner your medical status. If during the first date or discussion, you find yourself wanting to meet this person again, it would be wise to disclose your cancer diagnosis.

You may choose to be quite open about your prostate cancer status right from the beginning, such as one man we talked to. His strategy was to post a picture of himself at a public fundraising event for prostate cancer on his online dating profile. He found this to be an easy way to bring up his diagnosis.

If you find that after a couple of dates things start to progress with this new companion, and you feel hopeful that a relationship can develop, you may find it helpful to share more specific information about your treatment with that person. This would mean telling your companion what it is like to be on ADT. Consider sharing this chapter (or the next, "Impact on Committed Relationships") with that person as you are getting to know him or her. That would be a good way of helping your companion understand your experience as a prostate cancer patient. Also, because ADT may be affecting you not just sexually (e.g., changes in your emotional expression, energy level), you may also want to share information about these changes with that person. Our research shows that patients, partners, and friends, who are informed about how ADT affects men, all cope better, and remain more connected, than those who are not in tune with each other.

Some single men on ADT are hesitant to begin new relationships, not because of anxiety around disclosing their cancer history *per se*, but specifically in relation to their change in sexual function. The following chapter details the many ways in which men's sexual function may be altered, but also provides different strategies to promote sexual intimacy, despite changes in sexual function. If you are concerned about how to navigate new sexual or intimate relationships, this chapter should give you insights on how to adjust to changes, and how to involve new partner(s) in adapting to these changes.

Perhaps most importantly, do not focus exclusively on sexuality. We will discuss ways to build and maintain closeness and connection within relationships, even without sexual activity. It may be helpful to remember that you are not alone in dealing with changes in sexual function. Over half of men in their 70s and older, who do not have cancer, nevertheless report that they are no longer sexually active. Over two thirds of women report loss of sexual desire after menopause, which occurs between ages 48 to 55. Yet for these individuals close companionship is rewarding. It may be worth adding that this is true whether one's preference for partners is toward women or men.

It may feel different entering a new relationship, as many new relationships do have some focus on a sexual connection, but it is possible to find either (a) a partner who is not interested in sex or (b) a partner who is open to being sexual in ways other than typical penetrative intercourse. The bottom line is that ADT need not be a barrier to forming new and intimate relationships with others, be they of a sexual or nonsexual nature. But they will require openness and honesty.

Maintaining a Sexual Relationship

Note: This section is for patients and their partners who desire a sexual relationship. There is also some content in the text that follows on solo sexual activity (i.e., masturbation) without a partner. Read on if you want to learn more about strategies to stay sexual.

Some of the suggestions in the following discussion of sexuality may go beyond what you are comfortable with. We include explicit descriptions of sexual practices and activities. You may be surprised to learn that some couples continue to enjoy sex despite undergoing ADT. If you, too, desire to maintain sexual intimacy, you are encouraged to communicate openly with your partner to establish what you both are willing to try or not try. Proceed with an open mind.

Sexuality starts with how you feel about yourself overall. It is not just about your body parts. You may choose to express your sexuality in different ways: by the way you dress, by the way you groom yourself, by the way you carry yourself, by the ways in which you have sex, and whom you choose to have sex with. Sexuality, particularly with couples, usually includes caring for someone else intimately. The role that sexuality plays in your life is affected by many factors including age, environment, health, culture, beliefs, relationships, opportunities, and interests.

Testosterone is one thing that affects your sex drive and sexual performance, but it is not the only thing. Physical and psychological details, such as anxiety and weight gain, can also significantly affect how you view yourself and consequently how you perform sexually. It is important to consider how you view yourself and your partner, and make an effort to think positively about sex.

The brain has a major influence on sexuality. If you are anxious, worried, or depressed, it will be harder to be turned on by the thought of sex. Sometimes, it is easy to forget why sexual activities between you and your partner can be so beneficial. Some of the benefits are as follows:

- Provides an opportunity to be close and connected, both physically and emotionally.
- Increases blood circulation and releases muscle tensions.
- Releases hormones that help you relax.

> Some worry that becoming sexually aroused will raise testosterone levels and promote cancer growth. Be assured that this is NOT the case.

Suggestions for Enjoying Sensual Pleasure With Low Libido

Couples undergoing ADT often find that they can no longer rely on spontaneous sexual urges to spark physical intimacy because of the patient's reduced libido. Of course, independent of ADT, as individuals get older, spontaneous desire for sexual interactions usually declines, so changes in levels of desire and interest in sexual intimacy naturally change over the course and length of a relationship.

Although, as a couple, you may have been used to sexual spontaneity before starting ADT, this does not mean you have to give up on all sexuality. Sexual intimacy may still flourish if the setting is carefully prepared. Part of what makes a meal elegant is the planning that goes into it: opening a bottle of wine, putting on some nice music, and lighting candles. In a similar way, sensuality may be enhanced by planning the time and place for sexual intimacy. It also helps to be open-minded to exploring new things that you may not have done before, but be sure to plan together and communicate your ideas and expectations.

Be Flexible About Who Initiates Intimacy

One of the most important factors for maintaining physical intimacy after ADT is being flexible about who initiates sex. If the partner now has stronger sexual urges than the patient, the partner may need to take the lead in initiating physical affection. Being the initiator of physical intimacy may be a new and different experience for some partners. If the patient has typically been the initiator, being pursued may be new for him. For this shift in roles to work well for both individuals, both partners need to be clear on expectations, which means that you need to discuss your expectations with each other ahead of time. Discussing the feelings associated with asking one another to engage in physically intimate activities can help prevent misconceptions. Sometimes, initially, it helps to remove the expectation that starting pleasurable sensual activities must lead to intercourse or to orgasm. Removing this expectation helps to decrease any anxiety associated with the feeling that either of you has to "perform" as you did before ADT. Accepting such changes in the roles of who initiates sensual play can work for both partners—if they both communicate about expectations.

Redefine Your Sexual Activities

Often when people think of sex, they think specifically of penetrative intercourse. At the same time, many people also recognize that there can be much pleasure and sensuality in other forms of sexual interaction. It may represent a change from your focus before ADT, but try to approach sexuality with a focus on pleasure in a broad sense. Foreplay (i.e., the physical activity leading up to sexual intercourse) is an important part of sex and can be enjoyed even in the absence of intercourse (or orgasm) because of the closeness and attention your partner gives to you during this activity. Patients and partners can still enjoy nonpenetrative sexual activities. Experiencing enjoyable sexual activity on ADT requires an understanding that all encounters of pleasure and sensuality do not need to end with intercourse or orgasm. Each partner needs to understand how things have changed and be willing to give more attention to sensual touching, caressing, cuddling, and other aspects of sexual play. You may find that with a fresh approach to pleasure and sensuality you and your partner discover (or rediscover) ways of being intimate that meet each other's needs for physical affection.

With open discussion and conscious attention, activities focusing on pleasure and sensuality can be highly rewarding, and can build intimacy in ways that have been forgotten or have not been used before.

Many of the couples we met have shared with us that expanding their sexual life to include sensual touch, or sexual touch that does not necessarily finish with orgasm, has allowed them to begin to appreciate their partner in a new way. Sensual touch and caressing, as an alternative to very goal-oriented sexual touch with the objective of reaching orgasm or "using an erection before they lose it," can be a welcome change, and one in which partners feel truly valued for who they are as whole people, rather than focusing entirely on sexual behaviors.

A NOTE FOR GAY MEN ON ROLES

Many gay men admittedly have a preference for a sexual role during anal sex, that is, the penetrative ("top"), the receptive ("bottom"), or either role ("versatile"). Sexual problems due to prostate cancer treatments may impact these sexual practices. For example, many men who preferred being the penetrative partner have found that they need to take erection-enhancing medications after prostate cancer treatments. A man, of course, does not need erections to be the "bottom," but one described for us how being the bottom without erection can still be a challenge: "I still have the option of doing that [being receptive] and I don't even really need an erection for that, although it's not all that pleasurable."

(continued)

> Similarly it is possible to masturbate with a flaccid penis. As one man told us, "I can masturbate with a flaccid penis—but when you're having sex with somebody you need a bit more stimulation and having an erect penis is helpful."
>
> Some gay men who have ED from prostate cancer treatments have said, "Well, if I can't be a top, I can be a bottom." It is easy to make such a declaration—and sex role versatility is common in the gay world—but for some men the shift is neither natural nor easy. Among those who have switched roles, one who became a "bottom," reported to us, "I found my calling ... [and] ... reinvented myself as a bottom. There's been a lot more anal sex with me receiving since treatment, and my partner is happy with that." A key variable, of course, is the partners' preferred sex role and versatility.

Take the Focus Off Orgasm

Commonly, for a male with strong sexual urges the ultimate goal of a sexual encounter is orgasm, but with a reduced libido, it becomes more difficult for a man to achieve orgasms. This can become a problem for a man who stops making physical contact with his partner because he does not want to start anything he is not motivated to do, or does not feel capable of finishing. However, as mentioned earlier, it is essential for the person on ADT to realize that physical contact that does not lead to orgasm may still be vitally important for both him and his partner.

Be Aware of Decreased Responsiveness to Sexual Touch

ADT and the lack of testosterone are associated with decreased sensitivity to erotic touch. Therefore, as a man on ADT, you may not get the same genital pleasure or skin responses that you once did when a partner touched you. A patient in this situation needs to be aware that emotional and physical attention is a sign of his partner's caring. He must be careful not to simply reject this touch because it is not as sexually alluring as it may have been in the past. Sadly, those who ignore a partner's advances may hurt the partner, causing feelings of rejection. This may discourage further attempts to initiate physical intimacy, which can undermine intimacy overall and weaken a couple's bond.

Partners of patients on ADT need to know that lowered sex drive and limited responsiveness to sexual advances are *not rejections of them* as persons, partners, or lovers. Patients should be aware, however, that muted responses from them might be interpreted that way. Open discussion can help avoid the risk of the partner misconstruing a patient's low response to sexual stimulation as general rejection.

Enhancing Awareness of Sensation With Mindfulness Meditation

One way to cultivate awareness of sensations is to learn the practice mindful awareness. Mindful awareness, like other skills, is developed with practice. All too often we live our lives without being truly aware of our environment or what is going on in our bodies. Mindful awareness exercises help to develop the ability to focus on physical sensations in the body by turning your attention specifically to all that you can feel, see, hear, and smell. Specific instructions for how to practice a mindfulness-meditation exercise are presented in Chapter 5 on page 93. Initially, the mindfulness meditation exercise should be practiced on your own, and then you can introduce it into sexual activities with a partner. When using mindfulness during sexual encounters, you will practice to focus on what is happening in the body in response to sexual touch. During sexual encounters, rather than following distractions in thoughts and getting hung up on judgments or feelings about your sexual experience, you can train yourself to bring your attention fully to the physical sensations you are experiencing during each intimate encounter. Mindfulness practice has also been demonstrated to be an effective treatment for reduced sexual desire in women, but remains to be tested in men.

This type of exercise also helps to foster an appreciation for new experiences or types of sexual stimulation. It may even assist in helping you identify the types of stimulation that you do or do not like, as this can also change as a part of being on ADT. Practicing mindful awareness during sexual activity or sensual touch with your partner can help to promote increased awareness of physical sensations and touch. Conversely, increasing your ability to be aware of bodily sensations can improve enjoyment of sensual or sexual pleasure. When adding mindfulness meditation to sensual touch with your partner, you can follow the instructions we provided in Chapter 5, and practice them while lying down next to each other. Alternatively, you can have one partner focus on the sensations in the body while the other partner gently touches, and then take turns giving and receiving touch. You may start by focusing in on the breath, but then move your attention to the sensations of touch that your partner provides, or to the sensations of touch that you feel as you touch your partner.

Stimulate Your Sexual Appetite

The French axiom, *"L'appetit vient en mangeant,"* or *"Appetite comes while we eat,"* captures the concept of pleasure and sensuality without pressure for intercourse. It resonates with the experience of many couples, especially for those on ADT. Most of us have experienced a lack of an appetite for food; the

One woman said, "I bought some sexy underwear and … I just laid a path [of rose petals] through to the bedroom. It obviously didn't change his libido but it led to a lot of laughter and that seems to have been a huge missing factor."

mere idea of being expected to eat an entire four-course meal when we are not particularly hungry mutes our willingness to take the first bite. However, if we are gently invited to take a taste knowing that we can just nibble the bits that we find appealing and stop when we are full, we can often enjoy the food, and may even find that our appetite is stronger than we thought. Similarly, many men on ADT are more willing to engage in sensual touching when there is no pressure to reach climax or to engage in activities that do not seem appealing. To stay with the food metaphor, one can have a grand meal made up of only the most elegant appetizers without eating a main course. It is possible for a male with both ED and low libido to learn to enjoy sensuality, and sexual pleasure, without reaching an orgasm.

One way to stimulate the sexual appetite is to use erotic material. Erotic material comes in many forms: movies, books, short stories, poetry, music, magazines, works of art, and even educational programs. Erotic material often provides a good starting point to increase one's arousal or awareness of physical touch. Bear in mind that erotic material does not necessarily mean pornographic material. Pornography typically focuses on the visual representation of explicit sexual acts, while erotica is usually subtler and tends to imply sexual interest rather than explicitly show sex organs. Erotic material may or may not arouse a patient with a low libido, but even if it does not help him with arousal, watching or reading erotic material together may serve to draw partners closer together, and open them up to exploring new options.

There is an abundance of erotic material available on the Internet accessible via a Google search. Books can also be purchased with erotic stories/literature at your local bookstore—try searching the love, relationships, or sexuality sections. If you browse through them and find something that you are uncomfortable with, or that does not fit your taste, then skip it and select another. You may not know what you or your partner will find interesting or arousing until you try it.

Orgasms Without Ejaculation

If you had other treatments for prostate cancer before ADT, such as a radical prostatectomy or radiotherapy, you may have had an orgasm but with little or no ejaculation. If you have not had prior treatment for prostate cancer, you are likely to discover that without testosterone you produce little or no seminal fluid when you orgasm. Thus, even if you had a functioning prostate gland before, it will probably become inactive when you are on ADT.

The absence of ejaculate does not, however, necessarily mean that there can be no orgasm, just as the absence of an erection does not mean there can be no orgasm. An orgasm can be thought of as a pelvic sneeze. With sneezes, there is a buildup of tension followed by a release. Or the sneeze can be stifled and the tension can disappear on its own. While a normal sneeze in one's head releases facial tension, an orgasm releases sexual tension. We can have wet sneezes or dry sneezes—they feel different but both are unmistakably sneezes. Similarly, a person can have wet orgasms (with ejaculate) or dry orgasms (with no ejaculate).

Again, these will feel different, but both are orgasms. Some couples celebrate that dry orgasms mean less mess; for some partners, dry orgasms make oral sex more enjoyable. Admittedly, the loss of ejaculate upon orgasm can be bothersome for many men. As one told us, "I find, when you've ejaculated, it's just more complete than when you have dry ejaculation. Okay, it's just longer and it's more relaxed than with the dry ejaculation." The loss of ejaculation may make patients feel their orgasm seems less complete and may be seen as a loss by their partner as well.

Sex: Beyond Intercourse

Many men with a reduced ability to have erections and intercourse are worried that they will not be able to sexually satisfy their partner without penetration. Penetration and/or sexual intercourse are often seen as the essential part of sexuality for some couples. Yet sexual activity can be understood as the expression of erotic love and physical affection between two individuals for the purposes of sexual arousal, pleasure, or connection. It may involve a variety of acts, not just penile penetrative sex, and most couples include a variety of types of touching and caressing as part of their sex play.

Activities that we typically think of as foreplay—for example, sexual talk, kissing, hugging, cuddling, sensual touching, genital touching, and oral sex—can be pleasurable in and of themselves, and can also lead to orgasm. It is okay not to reach orgasm every time, or even at all, with sexual activity. That does not mean that sex has to be any less intimate or that it cannot be pleasurable. Sometimes, it is the pressure to reach orgasm that takes the pleasure out of sex.

> One patient told us: "Libido is the starting point. But the ultimate point in the encounter is the orgasm, and I can't achieve orgasms now no matter what I do. So that part is missing: The carrot at the end of the stick is gone. You might get the erection, but that [alone] doesn't lead to the orgasm. Nevertheless I still find sexual encounters rewarding despite the fact that they are different from before because I still enjoy being caressed and I love giving my wife pleasure."

When an erection problem makes normal penile penetration impossible, some couples give up on all sexual activity. Others continue to be sexual in other ways. Couples who have good communication skills and have used a variety of types of touch prior to ADT are more likely to have a rewarding sexual life without intercourse.

Provide reassuring messages to your partner about how you enjoy giving pleasure; being in the right mindset will put your partner at ease and improve the experience. If your partner feels uncomfortable, or senses that you are uncomfortable, the experience may be less enjoyable.

> Many men on ADT tell us they still enjoy intimate contact without erections and with a reduced libido, but often their experiences become less goal oriented. Sexual touch can still be pleasurable and enjoyable but sexual activity may look quite different after ADT.

Suggestions for Pleasing Your Female Partner

The majority of women say it is easier to reach orgasm when orally or manually stimulated than through intercourse.

Consider trying this. Kiss your partner's thighs and tummy, slowly working your way toward her genitals. The clitoris is located toward the top of the vulva, between the labial folds of skin and above the vaginal opening and urethra. It becomes engorged as a woman becomes aroused and is highly sensitive to stimulation; therefore, gently touching here can provide great pleasure. Try kissing the clitoris, and using your fingers to provide gentle stimulation in a circular motion. Try using your tongue in an up-and-down motion on the clitoris. Pay attention to your partner's response (e.g., changes in breathing, movement toward or away from you). Try asking your partner if what you are doing feels good, or if she might like softer or firmer pressure. You may want to try inserting a finger into the vagina while providing oral stimulation. Touching your partner's hips, waist, or breasts while providing oral stimulation is another option.

Suggestions for Pleasing Your Male Partner

Many men can reach orgasm with oral sex without having an erection.

One evening while you and your partner are on the couch or in bed, you may want to try this. First, take his hand and kiss his fingers. If he feels comfortable with that, take one of his fingers in your mouth and suck on it like a lollipop. You may see him getting aroused, or at least curious. If he seems to be enjoying this, consider going further. Unzip his pants and begin with kissing or licking the penis. When you feel ready, take the tip of his penis into your mouth. You may wish to try sucking on it, much like a vacuum. Communicate with your partner to find out what his preferences might be and where his hot spots are. If you are worried about ejaculate at orgasm, you need not; men who have had their prostates removed will not have any ejaculate at orgasm. Men on ADT, even if they still have their prostate, will also have no or very little ejaculate.

Using Sexual Aids and Sex Toys

It has become increasingly common for couples to include "sex toys" in their sexual activities, whether or not ED or changes in libido are affecting their relationship. Using sex toys may or may not be a new idea for you and your partner, but you may now use them in a different way. The use of such objects may help lengthen your sexual interaction by saving your energy since you will not have to stimulate your partner manually for as long. There are a variety of such sex toys available, including *vibrators*, which come in many sizes and for many purposes, and *dildos*, which are used for penetration. These are great options for adding sexual activities to your sexual repertoire beyond penile-vaginal intercourse.

> **Some men on ADT have told us that they discovered, to their surprise, that with stimulation to the penis through a vibrator, and with enough desire, they can reach orgasm, though they had previously thought it was impossible.**

You may be familiar with various sex toys, but in case you are not, the following is some basic information on them. The main feature of a vibrator, as the name suggests, is that it provides stimulation through vibration. There are vibrators designed specifically for men to place around the head of the penis where the nerve endings are most sensitive. Some products are relatively inexpensive, such as the Wahl® vibrator with the cup attachment. The Viberect®, which has double paddles, is specifically marketed for men with ED; however, it is very pricey, and there are no published data to show that it is superior to two simpler and cheaper vibrators used together. There are also vibrators designed so that the penis can be inserted, such as Cobra Libre from funfactory.com or Pulse from hotoctopuss.com. When a man uses such a device, the device can be placed on top of his partner's genitals, too. Thus, the vibration stimulates both partners.

> **Vibrators can be used to stimulate the genitals, perineum, and anal area. Those designed in the shape of a penis may be used for penetrative stimulation. They come in a variety of materials including silicone, metal, and glass. There is a device called the Aneros®, though not a vibrator, which was originally designed for prostate stimulation. The Aneros can be inserted into the anus to stimulate the prostate gland, and the person can move it by contracting the pelvic floor muscle. However, men without the prostate gland may also find pleasure from this device because it stimulates the erogenous peri-anal area as well.**

Only buy high-quality sex toys that are visibly new. Be sure to clean sex toys before each use. There is some concern about the chemicals in soft toys, so if you purchase them, consider covering them with a condom. If you have any allergies, such as to latex, ensure that your toys are hypoallergenic and that you do not use oil-based lubricants with them. You should not use a silicone

> One couple, with great hesitancy, decided to try an ED treatment we had recommended—something they had never done before. The partner reported back to us that while they found it was not for them, the process of experimenting with it led them both to giggle and laugh a lot together—and in the process they shared a new and intimate experience that made them feel closer to each other than before they had tried it.

lubricant with a silicone sex toy, as it will erode the toy. Do not be too rough with toys; be careful not to insert too deeply or forcefully.

Sexual Devices to Permit Insertive Sex Without Erections

An alternative to ED treatments is for a male to use an external penile prosthesis (more commonly known as a strap-on dildo) to penetrate his partner. A harness is worn on the man's hips, which holds a penis-like dildo in essentially the same position that an erect penis would be. When the partner reaches down and stimulates the patient's penis with a lubricated hand while the patient thrusts with the strap-on, some patients have reported that it feels exactly as if their penis is inside their partner and they were able to reach orgasm. Patients who have used such an external penile prosthesis report relief knowing that they do not have to fear losing an erection during sexual activity or disappointing their partner. Consequently, both patients and partners have reported that they enjoy this sexual aid. One company, SpareParts®, makes a harness specifically for males, called the Deuce®, which can be purchased in several different sizes from many of the larger sex shops in North America. For more information see https://lovelifeandintimacy.com/

> An experienced sales person at a popular sex shop told us that what she likes most about her job is that couples who come into the store are invariably curious and upbeat, never unhappy.

Patients may also consider exploring a penile sleeve or a penile support device for penetrative sex. A penile sleeve is made of plastic and comes in a shape of a penis but the inside is hollow. The penis can then be inserted into the sleeve. At least one company—the RxSleeve—manufactures a penile sleeve that can be attached on a harness too, similar to the harness for a strap-on dildo. A penile sleeve is available with different thicknesses. If you are interested in using one, you will need to find one with the right thickness. If you cannot get any erection, you may need to use the one with firm thickness, but if you have a partial erection, you might be able to use the medium thickness. There is also a penile support device that can be braced on a flaccid penis. At least one company—the Elator—designs their product so that it can brace the penile shaft and pull the glans away from the base of the penis. An instructional video on how to use this device can be found on: www.youtube.com/watch?v=AokWVYxpzY4.

The three options mentioned previously (i.e., external penile prothesis, penile sleeve, and penile support device) can be used regardless of how much erection you have. For example, even if you have a complete loss of erection, you may still be able to use them for penetrative sex. One positive thing about these options is that they are not as invasive as other erection treatment like a penile implant.

If the idea of sex toys is awkward for you, consider experimenting with simpler things. You can start out with massage oils, feathers, and other erotic touch products that you may not have used before; you can eventually experiment with a sexual aid such as a vibrator, and progress from there. The best way to approach the use of sex toys is to have an open mind and not be afraid to laugh if it does not go as well as you expected. Sometimes just experimenting with something new can bring men and their partners closer. Just talking about such options and shopping together (in stores or online) for sex aids can help build intimacy.

> **Some of the benefits of incorporating toys into your sex play may include experiencing excitement associated with trying something new and different, discovering the capacity for a new kind of penetrative intercourse (e.g., use of a hand-held or strap-on dildo), and avoiding fatigue during extended stimulation by using vibrators.**

Treatments for ED

ED is increasingly common as men age and is a common side effect of primary prostate cancer treatments (e.g., radiation, prostatectomy). The addition of ADT greatly increases the likelihood of ED. There are ways to restore the capability of having erections. However, the reduced libido of patients on ADT compounds the problem. Unfortunately, common ED treatments do not work for everyone—in particular for men on ADT. Attempting to find the best ED treatment can be a frustrating process and many couples give up on using them altogether.

Many men are reluctant to talk about the use of erectile aids, fearing that they will be seen as inadequate for relying on them, or even more inadequate if the aids do not work for them. Acknowledging the use of ED treatments can sometimes be helpful because it reveals honesty and openness, which can help to strengthen intimacy in a relationship. Remaining secretive regarding ED treatments may undermine trust and intimacy in the long run.

If you are not in a committed relationship, but have casual partner(s), you may be reluctant to disclose your use of an ED aid. However, this may also increase anxiety about performance and whether or not the aid will work. It might be helpful to acknowledge the use of the aid and the willingness to continue with other types of sexual activities (touch, oral sex) in the case that the aid fails to result in a full and firm erection. Being open about using an ED aid is better than leaving a partner to assume that the ED is due to a lack of interest, attraction, or arousal.

General Comments on Using Erectile Assistive Aids

While we believe that couples can have mutually satisfying sex without an erection, having an erection and penetrative sex may nevertheless be important for some patients and their partners. Some men find these strategies helpful and effective while others do not. Remember that if the strategy does not work, the failure is in the strategy, not you. It is important to keep an open mind and be willing to try different options, and at times retry some of those that may have failed in the past. If you decide to explore ED treatments there are many options available, ranging from the noninvasive (e.g., oral medication) to surgical interventions (e.g., penile implants).

With ED treatments you may find that

- The presence of an erection can help raise your own sexual interest.
- Your partner may become more aroused in the presence of an erection.
- You as a patient can enjoy pleasing your partner, even if you do not have the same quality of erection or orgasm.

But you may also find that

- The treatment simply does not work; most men on ADT find that common treatments for ED, in particular oral drugs, do not work well for them.

It is also possible that erections achieved through ED treatments may be disconcerting in the absence of sexual arousal. However, even if the experience is deemed unsuccessful, your partner may appreciate the effort and time you have taken to explore the options. This can help strengthen your bond as a couple. In other words, exploring new sexual styles and practices together can help maintain and even build intimacy, even if they do not exactly reproduce the experiences you had prior to prostate cancer treatments.

Whether or not you are planning to have sexual intercourse, some of the following treatments may prove helpful in restoring or improving erections.

Oral Medications

Oral medications for ED called **phosphodiesterase-5 inhibitors (PDE5i)**—Viagra®, Cialis®, Staxyn®, and Levitra®—are often the first line of treatment for ED; however, these drugs do not work as well when testosterone levels are low as they do when testosterone levels are in the normal range. The PDE5i medications need to be taken no less than 1 to 2 hours ahead of sexual activity. Sildenafil and vardenafil work over a 4- to 6-hour period. Tadalafil lasts in your system for up to 36 hours or more. While all of these PDE5i drugs can be taken daily, Cialis for daily use is formulated to maintain a steady level in your system so that you do not need to take a pill within an hour or two of engaging in sexual activity. These drugs have several side effects such as headaches, nasal congestion, and flushed face, which all go away when the drugs are stopped. These can cause discomfort though, and sometimes one brand will cause fewer side effects for you than another.

> **High-fat meals affect your body's absorption of Viagra, Staxyn, and Levitra. Do not eat a greasy, heavy meal, or you may find these pills do not work as well.**

PDE5i drugs can help maintain good blood circulation in the penis independent of their specific use in aiding sexual activity, but they are more effective when coupled with physical and mental sexual stimulation. These drugs do not increase libido or change ejaculation or orgasm; therefore, in order to see an erectile response, you must first engage in sexual stimulation. Sexual thoughts are usually not enough to generate an erectile response. PDE5i drugs also may not be very effective in men who have severe ED from either primary prostate cancer treatments or other diseases, such as diabetes.

PDE5i drugs should not be taken along with nitroglycerin (a medication for angina). They also are not recommended if you have

- Decreased liver or kidney function.
- Very low or high blood pressure.
- Recently had a heart attack or stroke.
- Certain eye disorders such as glaucoma.

It is important to discuss with your doctor whether a PDE5i drug, or any drug, is an option for you.

You can consume alcohol with these medications; however, you should be aware that alcohol itself often interferes with sexual ability.

Injections

Several medications can produce an erection when injected by a fine needle into one side of the shaft of the penis. These often work better for men on ADT than oral medications because they are not as influenced by testosterone levels and sexual arousal. Although initially hesitant to use this form of treatment, many men find that they are able to administer the injections successfully with high satisfaction and little discomfort.

The most commonly used injectable medication is prostaglandin E1 (also known as alprostadil, and available as Caverject®, Edex®, and Prostin VR®). Other drugs are also used; phentolamine and papaverine can be blended by a pharmacist to form a combination commonly called "bimix," which may also be effective. Utilizing all three drugs (prostaglandin E1, papaverine, and phentolamine) is sometimes called "Triple P" or "trimix."

In order to inject these medications, you need to have good visualization of the penis, so you may need a mirror or your partner to help. It helps to have an experienced healthcare provider teach you how to do the injections, as there is a precise way to do them that improves their effectiveness.

If you use injections for erections and have an erection that lasts for more than 3 hours, go to the emergency room (ER) right away. Although an ER visit under these circumstances may be embarrassing, erections that last more than a few hours can lead to permanent injury to the tissue in the penis from lack of oxygen. Most physicians suggest that injections should not be used more than three times a week.

> "I went into the exam room with a pretty high degree of apprehension, I mean, who really WANTS to stick a needle in the side of their penis? ... Looking down, I was in complete disbelief about what I was about to do. I was shaking a little, but I just did it. After a small bit of resistance it went right in! I was shocked that I felt almost nothing, it honestly felt like a mosquito bite."
> – JD1969, cancerforums.net

Intraurethral Suppositories

These small suppositories contain the medication prostaglandin E1 (sold as MUSE: Medicated Urethral System for Erection®). Instead of injecting the drug into the shaft of the penis, the MUSE system comes with a plastic applicator that places a small pellet of medication directly inside of the urethra. These suppositories are typically more effective when used with an elastic constriction ring (sometimes called a cock ring) that is placed at the base of the shaft of the penis in order to keep the blood contained in the penis. For anatomical reasons, intraurethral suppositories are typically not as effective as penile injections. Furthermore, using injections would require planning for sexual activities, and some men may be bothered by the loss of spontaneity.

Vacuum Pump

A vacuum erection device (VED) is a cylinder-shaped external pump that can be placed over the flaccid penis, using a lubricant to create a seal between the cylinder and the skin. These come with either a hand- or battery-powered pump that removes the air from the cylinder. This creates a vacuum around the penis. The lowered pressure draws blood into the shaft of the penis, making it swell and become firm. Once the penis is enlarged and firm, a constriction ring is slipped onto the base of the penis to retain the blood in the shaft of the penis. The pump can then be removed. Battery-operated pumps may work better if your hand dexterity is poor, but in general, the hand-operated pumps create a stronger vacuum. After the constriction ring is in place, it should only remain on for about 30 minutes. Rings left on for longer can damage the tissue of the penis. The VED can be used safely on a daily basis.

> **If you have a bleeding condition or are on blood thinners, such as Warfarin, penis rings and pumps are not recommended. They may increase your risk of bruising.**

A problem with erections produced by the VED is that only the shaft, and not the root of the penis, which lies inside the body, is engorged with blood. In natural unassisted erections, it is the engorged root of the penis that anchors the shaft and keeps the erection at the best angle for penetrative sex. Erections obtained with the VED, though firm, tend to "swivel" at the base. This is known as the "hinge effect." Patients and their partners should be aware of this hinge effect since penetrative sex with erections from the VED may require manual assistance for insertion and some adjustment of posture to prevent separation during intercourse.

Inflatable Penile Prosthesis

The Inflatable Penile Prosthesis (IPP) is a bionic system with inflatable cylinders surgically implanted into the shaft of the penis. The reservoir for fluid to fill the cylinders lies in the body cavity, and a small mechanical pump and valve lie in the scrotum. This hardware gives the man the option of having an erect penis for sexual activity and then a flaccid penis the rest of the time. The penis does not deflate after sexual activity until the man himself activates a release valve that lies in the scrotum and squeezes the fluid out of the cylinders. IPP devices are not visually detectable by others except for the small surgical scars where the hardware has been inserted. Once this procedure is done, it cannot be reversed. The IPP is an expensive option and is not always covered by insurance.

Solo Masturbation

Some men on ADT may also wish to masturbate alone. One patient indicated how he prefers to masturbate alone because he is embarrassed about his lack of erection: "I only masturbate alone as I am too embarrassed to be with a partner as I am unable to get an erection." Another patient mentioned how he uses sex toys for masturbation, "I live alone and do not have [partnered] sex very often. I use butt plugs, and cock rings for stimulation and excitement." However, without an erect penis, more intense stimulation of the penis may be needed to achieve sufficient erection. In the next section, we discuss how lubricant may facilitate masturbation when erection is absent.

> **"Since 2 years after treatment, I have changed my sexual practices whereby I give pleasure to myself exclusively by myself on average 3 times per week. This is always whilst bathing and/or showering and is almost always after use of a VED and a small dose of either Levitra or Viagra."**

> **One patient wanted us to note that, "anal stimulation while masturbating makes orgasm much more powerful [and he] enjoys all forms of anal stimulation."**

The Use of Lubricants for Men

With a full erection, stimulation of the sensory nerves in the penis is relatively easy (i.e., the nerves in the skin can be compressed against the firmer tissue below). However, without an erection, it is more difficult to stimulate those nerves. Consequently, to produce pleasurable feeling and arousal, more pressure and stimulation must be applied to the penis, and for a longer period of time. As a result, there can be irritation of the skin. This can be painful and distracting, so lubrication is essential to avoid discomfort during extended penile stimulation.

In this section, we provide information on the different types of lubricants. You are probably aware of the value of using lubricants, but in case you are not familiar, the following is a guide. In most drugstores and supermarkets, you can purchase lubricants that can be used for sexual activity. Some are warming, others are flavored, and others double as massage lotions.

- Water-based lubricants make for easier cleanup. Examples: K-Y® Liquid, Slippery Stuff®, Liquid Silk™, Astroglide®, or Dream Brands® The Natural. If using sex toys, a water-based lubricant is best for preserving the life of such products.
- Silicone lubricants are also available, and last longer. Sometimes they stain sheets and cannot be used with some sex toys.
- Some couples prefer to use natural products as lubricants, such as coconut oil or olive oil.
- Petroleum-based lubricants such as Vaseline® are **not** recommended because they can promote bladder infection.
- Clear, water-soluble, nonflavored lubricants are a good way to start.

Developing New Sexual Practices

Whether you are opting to try an erectile aid or shift your sexual activities to include nonpenetrative activities such as oral sex or the use of sexual toys, you are likely in for some changes to your sexual script. It is common to believe that we know what our partner wants, particularly if we have been together for many years. However, often what our partner wants and what we want changes over the years, and can even change from day to day. Some sexual activities, which may have once been very important to you, may not be as important now ... regardless of the influence of ADT. Similarly, you may think your partner is no longer interested in sexual activity when in fact your partner may still be in some ways. The more open and flexible you are to trying new sexual activities, the more likely you are to find options that work for you. You may also have to be persistent with these options, and try them more than once. You may even surprise yourself; activities you never predicted you would like, you may now enjoy.

How One Gay Couple Adjusted
"[With intra-cavernous injection], we could re-enter the bathhouse [for] multiple-partner play time. I felt [my partner] needed to have the choice to do that more than ever because he is a bottom and I was not performing the same. So we adapted with different sexual behaviors, practices, patterns, and activities."

Communicating about how important specific sexual activities are to each of you, and what you each find sensual and pleasuring, can help you recognize inaccurate assumptions or beliefs you may hold. This is an important step toward correcting those assumptions and achieving fulfilling intimate experiences.

Sometimes it is our beliefs and assumptions that keep us stuck and make it difficult for us to adapt.

Activity: Beliefs Awareness

Whether straight or gay, people often have unfounded beliefs about themselves and their sexual relationships. For example, a straight man may think that his partner will not be satisfied unless she is penetrated. A gay man who identifies as a "top" may assume that his "bottom" partner will leave him if he cannot sexually satisfy him through anal intercourse. These can be devastating assumptions for a man who is experiencing reduced libido and ED due to ADT. Similarly, if patients lose interest in sex, partners may assume that they are no longer loved or desired. Beliefs or assumptions such as these can leave men on ADT and their intimate partners feeling isolated and depressed.

As a first key step toward maintaining intimacy in the face of ADT, it helps to be aware of your assumptions and discuss them with your partner. Often confronting an assumption and then challenging it, or having your partner challenge it, can clarify what is truly going on.

Here are a few different examples:

1. Example of what a single man on ADT might be thinking:
   Belief
   Single patient: Who would want to be with a man who has no sexual interest?
   Challenging That Belief
   Single man: I can still give sexual pleasure and enjoy giving pleasure, even if I am not very turned on.

2. Example of what a partnered man on ADT might be thinking:
   Belief
   Patient: My partner may assume that I am not attracted to her or him if I cannot get a firm erection during sexual activities.
   Challenging That Belief
   Patient: If I reassure my partner that I am attracted to her or him, and tell her or him about my physical difficulties in getting an erection, he or she will not take my ED personally.
   Belief
   As a man, if I cannot have erections, I cannot satisfy another person.
   Challenging That Belief
   I can ask my partner what his or her needs are and how to please my partner in other ways, either physically or sexually; for example, through sensual touch, massage, or oral sex.

3. An example of what a man's partner might be thinking:
   Belief
   Partner: My partner (the patient) has no libido when around me because he no longer loves and desires me.
   Challenging That Belief
   Partner: My partner (the patient) may no longer become sexually aroused, but he still loves spending time with me. He likes being physically intimate with me, even if that intimacy is not sexual.

   Think of some beliefs that you may have about yourself, your relationship with your partner, or your relationship with others once the effects of ADT begin. Then challenge each belief in the following spaces provided. See the Appendix for an additional copy (p. 168).

Belief

_____
_____
_____

Challenging That Belief

_____
_____
_____

Belief

_____
_____
_____

Challenging That Belief

_____
_____
_____

Activity: Pros/Cons Table

If you have been reading through this book chapter by chapter, you should be familiar with the value of the Pros/Cons table by now. This exercise can be applied to any decision you are thinking about making in your life. Here is an example as it may relate to addressing sexual intimacy.

	PROS	CONS
MAKING THE CHANGE: Try engaging in nonpenetrative sexual activity	• Remain sexually connected with my partner • Provide pleasure to my partner • Enjoy receiving pleasure myself	• It might make me sad to compare what we used to have with what we can do now
STAYING THE SAME: Don't have sex until my erections come back	• Don't have to focus on what I have lost • Avoid feeling like a failure when I can't get an erection	• My partner and I may feel disconnected

Now, try it out for yourself.

	PROS	CONS
MAKING THE CHANGE:		
STAYING THE SAME:		

Activity: Action Plan

In the previous chapters, you were introduced to an Action Plan on page 34. Again, you are reminded that it is best to start small with something very manageable (e.g., arranging a date night) before you take on larger-scale goals (e.g., using an erectile aid for sexual intercourse). You may wish to place your Action Plan in a location where you will see it regularly throughout your day.

Action Plan Example: Increasing physical affection with my partner

What I plan to do: show my partner more physical affection

When I plan to do it: *give my partner a kiss and hug in the morning when I leave for work and when I get home; go to bed 10 minutes earlier than usual so we can cuddle in bed before we go to sleep*

Who I might do it with: *my partner*

Where I plan to do it: *in my home*

Why my plan is important: *to help my partner feel appreciated, loved, and prioritized*

What might get in the way: *forgetting*

How I will address what might get in the way: *I will tell my partner my plan so we will both be more affectionate with each other, which will remind me to put in the effort.*

Action Plan Example: *Getting out more*

What I plan to do: *go to a club to socialize and dance*

When I plan to do it: *Friday night*

Who I might do it with: *My friend Pat will probably go with me. Pat usually likes to go dancing.*

Where I plan to do it: *my favorite club*

Why my plan is important: *I need to be with people.*

What might get in the way: *getting too anxious*

How I will address what might get in the way: *Tell Pat that I am a bit anxious but I know it would be good for me to get out again, and could use the support.*

The following text has a blank copy that you can fill out. An additional copy is located in the Appendix (p. 162). It helps to be as specific as possible.

Action Plan: _____

What I plan to do: _____
_____

When I plan to do it: _____
_____

Who I might do it with: _____
_____

Why my plan is important: _____
_____

Where I plan to do it: _____
_____

What might get in the way: _____

_____

How I will address what might get in the way: _____

_____

Activity: Goal Setting and Confidence

In order to support your goal, take a moment to rate the following factors associated with your goal. First, write down your goal (this might be what you have written as an Action Plan):

GOAL #1 _____

i) Rate how confident you feel that you will achieve your goal:
   1   2   3   4   5   6   7   8   9   10
   Not confident   Very confident

ii) Rate how motivated you are to accomplish your goal:
   1   2   3   4   5   6   7   8   9   10
   Not motivated   Very motivated

iii) Rate how likely you are to actually carry out your goal:
   1   2   3   4   5   6   7   8   9   10
   Not likely   Very likely

If any of your answers are *less than five*:

- Some ways to enhance motivation: (a) Enlist the help of your partner to hold you accountable; (b) set up a reward system so that when you have achieved the goal, you can reward yourself; (c) review a list of the possible benefits that may come from this change in behavior.
- If your confidence rating is really low, consider revising your goal—is it too ambitious? Can you start with a more modest goal and work your way up to a more significant lifestyle change?
- If you are at a two, three, or four, for any of the questions, remind yourself of the reason you chose that number and not a zero—what are the reasons why you are motivated to make this change?
- Another strategy is to consider completing the previous Pros/Cons table to help you identify your motivations (pros) for making this change, but also some of the barriers (cons) that might be getting in the way of making the change.

Effects on Intimate Relationships and Sexuality: Essentials

ADT will probably influence the sexual and intimate aspects of your relationships. Most men (approximately 90%) on ADT experience a reduced libido, leading to less sexual desire, or even no desire, for sexual activities. Everyone reacts differently to these changes. It can be a source of relief for some couples and can cause significant distress for others. You may need to discuss what sex means to you and to your partner, and how the two of you will adjust to this change.

If you are single, changes in sexuality may lead to worrying about how you might navigate potential relationships in the future. Couples may want to explore together issues such as, "How might we maintain physical closeness, if sexual activity is no longer a prominent physical interaction between us?" Patients on ADT should expect a need to work to maintain sexual activity when they do not have spontaneous sexual desire to remind them to initiate sexual interactions.

Even with reduced libido, though, it is possible for some men to find sexual pleasure and sensuality. As a couple, you can redefine your sexual activities to include activities other than penile-dependent penetrative sex. You can explore new or forgotten sexual activities. The partner who, previous to ADT, may have been less responsible for initiation can become more expressive and be the one to initiate sensual activities. You can make the commitment to sample sensual and pleasurable activities without pressure to achieve erection, intercourse, or orgasm. The mere act of jointly planning the time and location for these activities can help maintain an intimate bond. Together, you can practice sensual touch or try activities to stimulate your appetite for physical intimacy and sensuality.

Gay relationships in particular take a real hit, where the ability to produce firm erections and ejaculate are sources of sexual self-esteem. Being open to explore new ways of being sexual (e.g., experimenting with receptive sexual experiences) can broaden opportunities to engage in sexual activity. Single individuals may need to draw on the support of friends and family in dealing with the changes associated with ADT, and in finding encouragement to continue to venture into the dating world. Individual sexual activity may still be valued when a person does not have a sexual partner, and these individuals may do well to explore new strategies to enhance sexual stimulation (e.g., using sex aids and toys, erotica, lubricants, etc.). Whatever your individual context, the specific exercises in this chapter may help you plan ahead and decide what is important to you.

Moving Forward: Questions for Discussion

Questions for Single Men:
- Who might understand what I am going through; who might I trust enough to share my feelings with?

- When I think of past lovers, who might have accepted me despite the effects of ADT?
- How comfortable am I in joining an online or face-to-face support group for gay men with prostate cancer?

Questions for Couples:
Starting conversations about sexuality is often difficult. The following questions for couples to ask each other may help to initiate communication and clarify expectations about sexual activities:

- Are you comfortable with one of us reaching orgasm even if the other does not?
- How do you feel about us touching, caressing, and cuddling without either of us reaching or attempting to reach orgasm?
- What do you think about us acquiring a sex toy to use in our sex play?
- Is there a better time for us to have sexual activity than waiting until the end of the day when we are tired?

The patient may want to ask his partner:

- What should we do when you get aroused and I do not?
- Is it okay if I bring you to orgasm through touching or oral caressing even though I no longer have full erections?
- How do you feel about us using or exploring erectile aids and/or sex toys?

The partner may want to ask the patient:

- Do you still enjoy me touching you even though you do not get fully sexually aroused?
- What kinds of touching do you most enjoy now?

NOTES:

_____

_____

_____

_____

Effects on Intimate Relationships and Sexuality

7

IMPACT ON COMMITTED RELATIONSHIPS

Couples may be at risk of experiencing deterioration in their relationship when the patient is on androgen deprivation therapy (ADT). One reason this can occur is that couples do not know how to communicate about the changes that are occurring within their relationship. Those who neglect to communicate with each other may feel isolated. Those who think they must hide their feelings and emotional changes, not only from their partner but also from others, may withdraw from friends and social networks.

Men who feel closest to their partners during sexual activity may withdraw from them when their sex drive is diminished by ADT. The couple may talk less because the patient no longer feels close to his partner. This can leave the partner feeling less wanted, less desired, and less attractive. These losses can be traumatic to each individual, and to the couple as a whole. For example, one patient told us: "Not having a good sex life really made me withdraw. I wasn't even going to touch her because she would think I would be interested when I'm really not, and then she might get all hot and bothered and I'm not…."

In sharp contrast, there are other couples who find that they actually connect more with each other because the experience of having cancer has brought them closer together. Some report that after many years together, they were perfectly fine with no longer having penetrative sex and yet were still able to maintain true intimacy in their relationship. In fact, our research confirms that better understanding among a couple, where the partner understands the emotional changes that a man experiences while on ADT, can actually help

> **Having a supportive partner has survival value.** For prostate cancer and several other cancers, it has been shown that having a supportive partner or spouse actually improves survival over and above cancer treatment. For certain cancers, and prostate is one of them, the median increase in survival that comes from having a partner exceeds the survival benefit of chemotherapy. For that reason alone, men on ADT who are currently in a relationship should make an effort to keep their partnership strong. The key to this is open communication and an appreciation of the individual needs of the patient and the partner.

preserve their emotional intimacy. Also, couples in which the patient is more physically active show better relational adjustment over the course of being on ADT. Couples who read this book and planned for adapting to sexual changes were also more likely to maintain sexual activity than those who did not. Therefore, the more engaged you are, together or "as a couple," in addressing the changes that can happen after starting ADT, the better it will be for your relationship.

Most people find it important to feel genuinely understood by their partner and to know they can talk about things, even things that stir up strong emotions. Initiating a discussion on emotionally sensitive topics can be challenging at first, but can help increase a couple's confidence that they can face whatever new challenges lay ahead. Yet, as the partner of an ADT patient describes in the following section, verbal communication is not the only way to share your feelings.

Potential Changes in the Relationship

Changes in the Way You Interact With Each Other

> "We take such comfort in [talking], yet we can undo everything we've said in one gesture or in one look, or even in one misinterpretation. Show me. Take me outside and let's watch the sunset together. Put your arm around me and pull me to your side for a long hug that tells me I'm treasured.... Touch me, even if it's just a gentle hand on my shoulder, or on my leg beneath the table ... ease off at the first sign of resistance. I will do the same, always respecting the signals you give, whether you utter them or not. Show me. Discover me. Rediscover us. Show me what you are saying is true. Then I'll listen to what you need to say."
> —Partner/caregiver as quoted in "Intimacy Challenged by Surgery, Radiation, or ADT" by Charles (Chuck) Maack (www.theprostateadvocate.com)

It is possible that during or after ADT, partners may change the ways in which they relate to each other, and even change the activities that they engage in together at home. Some couples dealing with cancer report being able to draw closer to each other, finding new appreciation for their relationship. Other couples dealing with ADT say that because they are unable to maintain a high level of sexual intimacy, they have started to drift apart; they live in the same house, but put on an act of being married. One or both partners may come to resent the other for the changes that are occurring in themselves and in their relationship. To better understand the impact of ADT in your own relationship, consider reflecting with your partner on the ways you relate to each other, and how your relationship may or may not change if you as a couple become less sexually active after beginning ADT.

Different couples respond to the changes brought on by ADT in various ways, and some couples find adapting to change easier than other couples. The following box presents one couple's story of drifting apart.

> **"The problems were solved when one day I moved into another room. I have my own bathroom, and I take care of my own affairs without involving my wife. It isn't the way I thought things would turn out, but it's preferable to endless quarrels and divorce, and my wife seems to be content.... We discuss practical matters without drifting into feelings, and when friends and family visit we put on a performance of intimacy and unity."**
> —Prostate cancer patient, as quoted in Navon and Morag, 2003

We hope that you can avoid ending up like this couple. The goal in bringing this story to your attention is to encourage you as a couple to think about and discuss ways to reduce the stress from ADT so you can remain close to each other and avoid drifting apart.

Differences in Coping Style

When conflicts arise around adapting to ADT, it is often because the patients and partners have different coping strategies. One may not want to dwell upon problems that they cannot easily solve. The other may feel better after talking over a problem, even if they do not see a simple solution. The first step to avoid having competing coping strategies lead to conflict in the relationship is to recognize that you are each using different coping strategies. Acknowledging these different styles is important, but that alone does not solve the problem. It may be necessary to take turns trying out each other's coping style, even though it will make you feel uncomfortable. For example, the person whose preference is open discussion may sometimes need to "let go" of more minor issues without discussion. On the other hand, if issues are of such significance that they cannot be "let go," it may be necessary to set aside a limited time for conversation (say 10 minutes) respecting that the communication is important, but also distressing for the partner who prefers avoiding discussion when no solutions are apparent. Compromising to accommodate each other's coping style from time to time can keep a couple's relationship strong when coping with cancer.

Increased Self-Doubt

Both the patient and his partner may experience increased self-doubt or decreased confidence when faced with the changes that ADT introduces to their lives. Either person may begin to question if their partner still sees him- or herself as attractive and desirable. Most people feel confident and attractive when they are able to sexually arouse their partner—and this could become an issue when ADT leads to reduced libido. The partners of patients in couples that were sexually active before he started ADT need to understand that the patient may not look at his partner in the same sexual way he did before ADT. However, the patient himself may not notice this change. Unfortunately, this may make the partner feel less sexually attractive, so it is important for partners to understand that the patient is not doing it on purpose, but it can be due to the psychological impact of ADT.

> **It is important to recognize that a man on ADT is less likely to spontaneously touch his partner, and that this can be devastating to the partner.**
>
> **You can do simple things to let your partner know that you still care and find your partner desirable. Make a point of telling your partner directly that you find your partner attractive and desirable. Do special things for each other (e.g., make a meal, write a love letter) that express how you feel. Spending quality time together and making a conscious effort to maintain physical contact and sensuality can help both of you overcome self-doubt and avoid drifting apart.**
>
> **Increased effort to display physical but nonsexual affection, and letting your partner know in visible ways that you care for your partner, can help to make up for and even overcome reduced sexual activity.**

Bear in mind that attraction and desire are not limited to sexual activities. We encourage you to openly reaffirm to each other that you appreciate each other's company, closeness, and intimacy, both of a sexual and a nonsexual nature.

If you neglect to do this, you or your partner may withdraw from the relationship and your communication and intimate bond might be damaged. If you doubt yourself and your relationship, it may make the transition to living with ADT, and managing ADT side effects in particular, even more challenging. Therefore, after the patient begins ADT, it is important that each of you make a concerted effort to let your partner know that you still care about the relationship and desire closeness, even if spontaneous and unassisted penetrative sex is no longer possible.

> "We show each other affection; we're cuddling and having our kisses. We're just there for each other ... we do love each other. We have our hugs. We have our laughs."
>
> —Adam, patient

One patient told us that he made his partner feel special by doing things that required some sacrifice on his part. He shared, "I love to make cabbage rolls for my partner even though I don't like to eat them myself."

Following are some of the things we hear from couples about why physical affection in general, and not just penetrative sex, is important to them. You may find some comments here that apply to you. Feel free to add your own thoughts to the list.

Physical affection with my partner:

- Calms me down
- Helps me feel special
- Makes me feel desired
- Helps me feel close to my partner
- Reminds me that my partner is here for me

_____

_____

_____

Activity: Pros/Cons Table

If you have been reading previous chapters of this book, you should be familiar with the value of the Pros/Cons table by now. This exercise can be applied to any decision you are thinking about making in your life. Here is an example as it may relate to addressing sexual intimacy.

	PROS	**CONS**
MAKING THE CHANGE: Show more physical affection to my partner	• Physical affection helps my partner to feel appreciated • Hugs and kisses keep us physically and emotionally connected	• Requires effort to remind myself to show her more affection • Might feel artificial
STAYING THE SAME: Stop being physically affectionate	• Prevents a misunderstanding that my partner might think I am interested in sex when I am not	• We may become more disconnected • My partner might interpret my lack of physical affection as not being interested

Now, try it out for yourself.

	PROS	CONS

MAKING THE CHANGE:

STAYING THE SAME:

Activity: Action Plan

In the previous chapters you were introduced to the value of an Action Plan. Again, you are reminded that it is best to start small with something very manageable (e.g., walking regularly) before you take on larger scale goals (e.g., running a 10-km race). Hang your completed form somewhere where you will see it every day, like next to your bathroom mirror or on your fridge, to remind yourself of your commitment to this goal.

Action Plan Example: Communicate More Effectively With My Partner

What I plan to do: have a conversation about ADT-related changes that might impact our relationship

When I plan to do it: Sunday morning when we go for breakfast

Who I might do it with: my partner

Where I plan to do it: at the local café and deli

Why my plan is important: to make sure that we talk about things explicitly to prevent misunderstandings and prevent avoidance of discussing important topics due to discomfort

What might get in the way: anxiety about the conversation

How I will address what might get in the way: I will tell my partner, so he or she can appropriately support me

Here is a blank copy that you can fill out. An additional copy is located in the Appendix on page 162. It helps to be as specific as possible when you are making your Action Plan.

Action plan:

What I plan to do: _____

_____

When I plan to do it: _____

_____

Who I might do it with: _____

_____

Where I plan to do it: _____

_____

Why my plan is important: _____

_____

What might get in the way: _____

_____

How I will address what might get in the way: _____

_____

Activity: Goal Setting and Confidence

A strategy that can help you in accomplishing your goal is to take a moment to rate the following factors: confidence, motivation, and predicted likelihood of completion. First, write down your goal (this may be what you wrote in your Action Plan):

Goal: _____

i) Rate how confident you feel that you will achieve your goal:
   1   2   3   4   5   6   7   8   9   10
   Not confident   Very confident

ii) Rate how motivated you are to accomplish your goal:
   1   2   3   4   5   6   7   8   9   10
   Not motivated   Very motivated

iii) Rate how likely you are to actually carry out your goal:
   1   2   3   4   5   6   7   8   9   10
   Not likely   Very likely

If any of your answers *are less than five*:

- Consider either enlisting the help of a friend to hold you accountable or implementing a reward system to help motivate you (see pages 57–58 for additional information on motivation, lapses, relapses, rewards, and support);
- Consider ways to enhance motivation, such as enlisting the help of your partner or a friend to hold you accountable or rewarding yourself with something you are looking forward to (Note: In the previous example the Action Plan involves having a discussion with a partner—a way to build in a reward may be to have that discussion at your favorite restaurant). For additional details regarding enhancing motivation and rewards see pages 57 to 58 in Chapter 3;
- Consider revising your goal—is it too ambitious? Can you start with a more modest goal and work your way up to a more significant lifestyle change? (Note: In the previous example the Action Plan involves having a discussion with a partner—it may be less ambitious to tackle a specific topic (e.g., sexuality or mood) rather than trying to discuss everything at one time);
- Remind yourself of the reasons why you are at a two, three, or four, and not a zero—what are the reasons why you indicated that you were not at a zero?
- Consider completing the previous Pros/Cons table. This will help you identify your motivations (pros) for making this change, but also some of the barriers (cons) that might be getting in the way of making the change.

Impact on Committed Relationships: Essentials

Individuals and couples react differently to the effects of ADT. Some couples will grow closer, and some couples will grow apart. Some couples may take on a role more like roommates rather than lovers. If it is of value for you as a couple to maintain the quality of the relationship you currently have, then you will have to plan ahead, preparing to adapt to changes. However, each of you will react in your own way, so it is important to communicate openly about how you are feeling.

As the man's libido decreases with ADT and the nature of sexual contact is altered, self-doubt may occur. For example, you may wonder if your partner still finds you desirable or attractive, either in sexual or nonsexual ways. The danger of this is that you as a couple can fall into a trap of self-doubt, where one or both of you isolate yourselves, and you fail to communicate with each other. This further fuels self-doubt and compromises your relationship. It is important that you frequently let each other know, even in little and nonsexual ways, that you still care for and desire each other.

Moving Forward: Questions for Discussion

The following are questions that can be helpful for partners to answer together:

- How do cancer and its treatments change the plans we had for our lives?
- How do we deal with the uncertainty of our future?
- In what ways do you feel different about me or yourself as a man/woman (e.g., abilities, roles, or dreams) now that we are facing a new cancer treatment?
- What have we lost—and what have we gained—through this experience so far?

Add your own questions here:

_____
_____
_____
_____

Then consider the following:

- How can I make sure that I let my partner know that I still love, desire, and cherish him/her even if ADT challenges our relationship?
- What are the things that make my partner feel most loved?
- What are the things that make me feel most loved?

NOTES:

_____
_____
_____
_____
_____
_____

8

UNIQUE CONSIDERATIONS FOR GAY RELATIONSHIPS

We recognize that gay men can have a wider variety of relationships than heterosexual men. A gay man may be in a long-term committed monogamous relationship with one partner or he may have nonmonogamous sexual relationships with others as well. There is a wealth of possible intimate relationships among the gay population that do not match the heterosexual model of "man and wife." Indeed, some gay men like being single and do not desire a committed relationship at all. We know that the loss of erection and reduced libido associated with androgen deprivation therapy (ADT) can make it particularly challenging for gay men to maintain a long-term relationship or to establish a new relationship, be it a casual or a committed one.

An all too common problem for men in general is that loss of sexual function (e.g., low libido, erectile dysfunction [ED]) can affect one's confidence in being able to start and maintain a new relationship. For example, one gay man stated, "I've lost all confidence that I could try [to be in a relationship] with anyone. I've gotten older. I've gotten uglier. I've gotten fatter. I've gotten flabbier. It's just in my head; that's the way it is."

The sexual changes themselves, such as the reduced amount of ejaculate, may affect your sexual experience. Furthermore, with ED, your ability to be the "top" in anal sex could be compromised, but you may consider using some sexual aids discussed in Chapter 6 to overcome this.

One important change with ADT is that spontaneous sex is lost because of reduced libido and ED. To remain sexual with a partner, you may need to schedule time for sex, particularly when preparation is needed ahead of time to use sexual aids. If you want to explore new sexual aids, we recommend that you and your partner discuss them ahead of time, and decide on what you want to try.

The problems generated by ADT can be particularly challenging for gay men who prefer noncommitted relationships, but make friends through sexual encounters. One patient described how he started to withdraw from his acquaintances, "I have distanced myself, or withdrawn to some degree from a number of relationships—a number of acquaintances. I've isolated myself, a little bit." Another one expressed his difficulty in forming new friendships, "We [in the past] used our sexual activity to make friends. That's the old way. I've had to learn a new way of making friends."

If you are not in a committed relationship now but are seeking such a relationship, we encourage you to be open and candid about your prostate cancer history when you meet new men. In particular, we encourage you to be honest about how prostate cancer treatments have affected your sexual function and desire. Having erectile difficulties may deter some men from getting involved in a relationship. We recognize that entering a dating scene can be an overwhelming and scary experience when you have sexual problems. You may also be unsure of when, how, and where to disclose your cancer history and sexual issues to a potential new partner. But being open and honest may provide a better chance of developing a genuine, cosupportive relationship in the long run than being forced to reveal sexual difficulties later or having a new partner discover it without any forewarning.

Without knowing about your prostate cancer treatment side effects, a new sex partner may be confused during a sexual encounter. For example, one patient told us about his experience with a new person, "'Why is this guy not getting an erection?' When we're playing around with each other, you know, they thought 'Maybe he's not that interested in me or something.'" Acknowledging cancer and sexual issues to a potential sex partner can be challenging for many men because this requires, at some level, accepting for themselves their situation and limitation. Understandably, many men are reluctant to reveal personal aspects of their medical history to people they do not know well. As with outing oneself in general, there is no simple formula for when or how to do this. Each new relationship has to be assessed separately. However, if there is a desire for and a hope for a long-term relationship the fact is that honesty helps build intimacy and, thus, strong partnerships.

ADT May Impact Committed Relationships for Gay Men

Both patients on ADT and their partners in stable relationships nevertheless report finding it difficult to communicate about the changes that are occurring within their relationship. Couples who neglect to communicate with each other can become isolated in their relationship. Men who feel they must hide their feelings and emotional changes may withdraw from friends and social networks in general.

Men who feel closest to their partners during sexual activity may withdraw from them when their sexual interests are diminished by ADT. Men may talk less because they no longer feel emotionally close. These losses can be traumatic for both the patient and the partner, and to the couple as a unit. Furthermore, patients may not look at the partners in a sexual way anymore, which may result in the partners feeling unattractive.

We have found, though, that some couples, both gay and straight, actually become more connected while the patient is on ADT because the experience of having cancer has brought them closer together. Yet again, communication is key.

We encourage those who are currently partnered to discuss ADT's impact with your partner as a way to remain close and avoid drifting apart. Even if sexual activity is diminished, it is beneficial to make the conscious effort to let your partner know that you find him attractive and desirable. This can be through displays of physical though nonsexual affection. Small acts of affection can help compensate for reduced sexual activity.

It is important that each of you make a concerted effort to let your partner know that you still care about him and desire closeness, even if spontaneous erections are no longer possible.

Increasingly we hear from couples both gay and straight about why physical affection in general, and not just sexual activity, is important to them in the face of ADT. But it takes conscious efforts from both patients and their partners.

Activity: Pros/Cons Table

If you have been reading previous chapters of this book, you should be familiar with the value of the Pros/Cons table by now. This exercise can be applied to any decision you are thinking about making in your life. Here is an example as it may relate to addressing sexual intimacy.

	PROS	CONS
MAKING THE CHANGE: Show more physical affection to my partner	• Physical affection helps my partner to feel appreciated • Hugs and kisses keep us physically and emotionally connected	• Requires effort to remind myself to show him more affection • Might feel artificial
STAYING THE SAME: Stop being physically affectionate	• Prevents a misunderstanding that my partner might think I am interested in sex when I am not	• We may become more disconnected • He might interpret my lack of physical affection as not being interested in him

Now, try it out for yourself.

	PROS	CONS
MAKING THE CHANGE:		
STAYING THE SAME:		

Activity: Action Plan

In the previous chapters you were introduced to the value of an Action Plan. Again you are reminded that it is best to start small with something very manageable (e.g., walking regularly) before you take on larger scale goals (e.g., running a 10-km race). Hang your completed form somewhere where you will see it every day, like next to your bathroom mirror or on your fridge, to remind yourself of your commitment to this goal.

Action Plan Example: Communicate More Effectively With My Partner

What I plan to do: have a conversation about ADT-related changes that may impact our relationship

When I plan to do it: Sunday morning when we go for breakfast

Who I might do it with: my partner

Where I plan to do it: at the local café and deli

Why my plan is important: to make sure that we talk about things explicitly to prevent misunderstandings and prevent avoidance of discussing important topics due to discomfort

What might get in the way: anxiety about the conversation

How I will address what might get in the way: I will tell my partner, so he can appropriately support me.

Here is a blank copy that you can fill out. An additional copy is located in the Appendix on page 162. It helps to be as specific as possible when you are making your Action Plan.

Action Plan:

What I plan to do: _____

_____

When I plan to do it: _____

_____

Who I might do it with: _____

_____

Where I plan to do it: _____

_____

Why my plan is important: _____

_____

What might get in the way: _____

_____

How I will address what might get in the way: _____

_____

Activity: Goal Setting and Confidence

A strategy that can help you in accomplishing your goal is to take a moment to rate the following factors: confidence, motivation, and predicted likelihood of completion. First, write down your goal (this may be what you wrote in your Action Plan):

Goal: _____

i) Rate how confident you feel that you will achieve your goal:
   1   2   3   4   5   6   7   8   9   10
   Not confident   Very confident

ii) Rate how motivated you are to accomplish your goal:
   1   2   3   4   5   6   7   8   9   10
   Not motivated   Very motivated

iii) Rate how likely you are to actually carry out your goal:
   1   2   3   4   5   6   7   8   9   10
   Not likely   Very likely

If any of your answers *are less than five*:

- Consider ways to enhance motivation, such as enlisting the help of your partner or a friend to hold you accountable or rewarding yourself with something you are looking forward to (Note: In the previous example the Action Plan involves having a discussion with a partner—a way to build in a reward may be to have that discussion at your favorite restaurant). For additional details regarding enhancing motivation and rewards see pages 57 to 58 in Chapter 3;
- Consider revising your goal—is it too ambitious? Can you start with a more modest goal and work your way up to a more significant lifestyle change? (Note: In the previous example the Action Plan involves having a discussion with a partner—it may be less ambitious to tackle a specific topic (e.g., sexuality or mood) rather than trying to discuss everything at one time);
- Remind yourself of the reasons why you are at a two, three, or four, and not a zero—what are the reasons why you indicated that you were not at a zero?
- Consider completing the previous Pros/Cons table. This will help you identify your motivations (pros) for making this change, but also some of the barriers (cons) that might be getting in the way of making the change.

Unique Considerations for Gay Relationships: Essentials

Individuals and couples react differently to the effects of ADT. When in committed relationships, some couples grow closer, and some couples grow apart. If it is of value for you as a couple to maintain the quality of the relationship you currently have, then you need to acknowledge the impact of ADT in order to adapt to it. However, each of you will react in your own way, so it is important to communicate openly about how you understand the way ADT impacts on you both directly as a patient and indirectly as a partner.

Given that relationships for gay men can be diverse (monogamous and committed, nonmonogamous but committed, noncommitted, casual, etc.) the sexual changes associated with ADT have a variety of impacts. As a man's libido decreases with ADT and the nature of sexual contact is altered, self-doubt may occur. For example, when sexual activity is threatened, you may wonder if your partner or new potential partners find you desirable or attractive, both in sexual and nonsexual ways. In a coupled relationship, either partner can fall into a trap of self-doubt when sex drive and sexual function are impaired. This can lead to withdrawal and compromises the relationship. It is important that you demonstrate even in little and nonsexual ways that you still care for and desire each other. ADT can also be challenging when you are single and looking to begin new relationships, be they long term or of a more casual nature. Take a moment to review the content in the Chapter 7 that provides guidance for open communication about ADT-related side effects when beginning new relationships. The advice there is applicable to both gay and straight men.

Moving Forward: Questions for Discussion

The following are questions that can be helpful for partners to answer together:

- How does cancer and its treatment change the plans we had for our lives?
- How do we deal with the uncertainty of our future?
- In what ways do you feel different about me or yourself as a man (e.g., abilities, roles, or dreams) now that we are facing a new cancer treatment?
- What have we lost—and what have we gained—through this experience so far?

Add your own questions here:

_____
_____
_____

Then consider the following:

- How can I make sure that I let my partner know that I still think he is hot, even if ADT challenges our relationship?
- What are the things that make my partner feel most loved?
- What are the things that make me feel most loved?

NOTES

_____
_____
_____
_____
_____

9

CONCLUSION: STAYING HEALTHY

As you come to the end of this book, we want to reiterate some of its major themes. We began by covering the rationale for a prostate cancer patient going on androgen deprivation therapy (ADT). Androgens stimulate prostate cell growth; thus, removing androgens or blocking their ability to attach to prostate cells can slow the growth of prostate cancer. We then covered the major drugs used to lower the level of testosterone in the body as well as drugs that block androgen's ability to stimulate prostate cancer cell growth. This can control the cancer for months to years, and in some cases decades.

ADT, however, has substantial side effects that can negatively impact a person's quality of life. We reviewed those side effects and strategies for overcoming them to maintain your health and quality of life. As you have read, there are both physical and psychological side effects of this treatment. Some of the side effects, such as reduced libido, impact not just the patient but also the dynamic of a couple's relationship. Managing ADT side effects can thus be a challenge for both the patient and those close to him.

Adapting to ADT and staying healthy while androgen-deprived can be best handled by both the patient and his loved ones being aware of the side effects and preemptively taking actions to deal with them. Some effects of ADT are very noticeable to patients (e.g., hot flashes, fatigue), but others are less obvious (e.g., osteoporosis, metabolic syndrome) yet potentially serious. Therefore, patients on ADT need to be carefully monitored by their physician to make sure the drugs are working and the more serious side effects are avoided or controlled.

Managing the physical side effects may require changing one's lifestyle (i.e., one's diet and exercise regime). Maintaining a healthy

BMI (body mass index) and an active lifestyle may not be easy, but the benefits are well established and they are the most effective way to stay healthy while on ADT. Based on what we know from research on goal setting and making lifestyle changes, we have included in each chapter activities and questions to assist you with making healthier changes in your lifestyle. You can refer back to those sections of the book at any time.

To deal with the psychological effects of ADT, particularly those that may be noticed by those closest to the patient, it helps to be aware of them and be willing to talk about them with others. Trying to hide or deny them is helpful for neither the patient nor those he normally interacts with closely. Remember that for those who are in intimate relationships, when the partner better understands the emotional changes (positive or negative) that the patient is experiencing, the couple appears to have a better relationship.

Sexuality is an important part of life for many men and their partners, and many patients give high priority to being able to be sexual despite prostate cancer treatments. We acknowledge that everyone has different sexual values and may place greater or lesser emphasis on sex depending on other factors in their lives, such as age, health status, and relationship status. For individuals who cherish maintaining some sexual activity, efforts can be made to redefine and thus recover rewarding sexual practices even for men on ADT. But this takes effort and an openness to explore new practices by both patients and their partners.

Single patients who wish to start a new relationship are encouraged to discuss their cancer and sexual issues with potential partners early in their relationship to avoid future conflicts. This is predicated on the fact that honesty and open communication are crucial in maintaining a good relationship in the long term.

For those who are no longer interested in being sexually active, but who are still in an intimate relationship, it may be helpful to ensure your partner feels the way you do. For couples who have stopped being sexual, it may also be wise to make efforts to maintain general nonsexual physical affection and good communication with each other in order to enhance intimacy in the relationship.

APPENDIX

In this appendix you will find additional copies of these tools for change:

1. Drug chart
2. Prostate-specific antigen (PSA) chart
3. Hot flash diary
4. Pros/cons table
5. Action Plan
6. Goal setting and confidence
7. Side effects self-assessment
8. Screening for emotional distress mood questionnaire
9. Beliefs awareness exercise

Appendix

1. Drug Chart

This chart can be used to document your specific medications for androgen deprivation therapy (ADT). For example, you might list the medication that you receive for your injections and how often you get your injection.

Medication	Dose and Starting Date	How Often?

2. Prostate-Specific Antigen (PSA) Chart

This is a chart for you to use to track your PSA results.

Date	PSA Level	Date	PSA Level	Date	PSA Level

PSA, prostate specific antigen.

3. Hot Flash Diary

This exercise will help you cope with bothersome hot flashes. The instructions for how to complete this exercise can be found on pages 20 to 21.

Day	Intensity (0–10)	Duration	Distressing Thought/ Appraisal	Coping Statement
Sunday				
Monday				
Tuesday				
Wednesday				
Thursday				
Friday				
Saturday				

4. Pros/Cons Table

Sometimes, even though you *want* to make a lifestyle change, you may need to persuade yourself that the change is in fact worthwhile. A pros/cons table is a great way to convince yourself, and you can redo it anytime you feel as if your life and priorities have shifted.

	PROS	CONS
MAKING THE CHANGE:		
STAYING THE SAME:		

5. Action Plan

Throughout the book there are suggestions for changes that will help you and your partner maintain a high quality of life while on ADT. An Action Plan is a structured way to help you be clear about your goals, and increase the likelihood that you will follow through on your plans.

Here are some blank copies that you can fill out. It helps to be as specific as possible when you are making your Action Plan. Specific examples are detailed in each chapter.

Action plan: _____

What I plan to do: _____

_____

When I plan to do it: _____

_____

Who I might do it with: _____

_____

Where I plan to do it: _____

_____

Why my plan is important: _____

_____

What might get in the way: _____

_____

How I will address what might get in the way: _____

_____

6. Goal Setting and Confidence

In order to support your goal, it can be helpful to ask yourself how confident you are that you can be successful in making this change.

First, write down your goal:

Goal: _____

(e.g., to start walking every day)

i) Rate how confident you feel that you will achieve your goal:
   1   2   3   4   5   6   7   8   9   10
   Not confident   Very confident

ii) Rate how motivated you are to accomplish your goal:
   1   2   3   4   5   6   7   8   9   10
   Not motivated   Very motivated

iii) Rate how likely you are to actually carry out your goal:
   1   2   3   4   5   6   7   8   9   10
   Not likely   Very likely

If any of your answers *are less than five*:

- Consider enlisting the help of your partner or a friend to hold you accountable;
- Consider revising your goal—is it too ambitious? Can you start with a more modest goal and work your way up to a more significant lifestyle change?
- Remind yourself of the reasons why you are motivated to make this change.

Appendix

7. Side Effects Self-Assessment

For descriptions and management strategies of the side effects in the following list, see the appropriate chapter.

1. *During the past month*, how often have you experienced hot flashes? (*Please circle one number.*)
   (1) More than once a day
   (2) About once a day
   (3) More than once a week
   (4) About once a week
   (5) Rarely or never

2. *During the past month*, how often have you had breast tenderness/sensitivity? (*Please circle one number.*)
   (1) More than once a day
   (2) About once a day
   (3) More than once a week
   (4) About once a week
   (5) Rarely or never

3. *During the past month*, have you noticed any breast enlargement? (*Please circle one number.*)
   (1) None
   (2) Minimal
   (3) Substantial
   (4) Moderate

4. *During the past month*, how much has your weight changed, if at all? (*Please circle one number.*)
   (1) Gained 5 lb./2.3 kg or more
   (2) Gained less than 5 lb./2.3 kg
   (3) No change in weight
   (4) Lost less than 5 lb./2.3 kg
   (5) Lost 5 lb./2.3 kg or more

5. *During the past month*, have you noticed a change in the amount of hair on your arms, legs, and torso? (*Please circle one number.*)
   (1) Loss of body hair on arms, legs, and/or torso
   (2) No loss of body hair

6. *During the past month*, how concerned have you been about changes in how your penis and scrotum look? (*Please circle one number.*)
   (1) Not concerned at all
   (2) A little concerned
   (3) Moderately concerned
   (4) Highly concerned

7. *During the past month*, how has your level of sexual desire been? (*Please circle one number.*)
   (1) Very low to none
   (2) Low
   (3) Moderate
   (4) High
   (5) Very high

8. *During the past month*, how has your ability to have an erection been? (*Please circle one number.*)
   (1) Very poor to none
   (2) Poor
   (3) Fair
   (4) Good
   (5) Very good/excellent

9. *During the past month*, how often have you experienced a problem remembering something that you thought you knew well? (*Please circle one number.*)
   (1) More than once a day
   (2) About once a day
   (3) More than once a week
   (4) About once a week
   (5) Rarely or never

10. *During the past month*, how often have you felt sad or depressed? (*Please circle one number.*)
    (1) More than once a day
    (2) About once a day
    (3) More than once a week
    (4) About once a week
    (5) Rarely or never

11. *During the past month*, how often have you felt a lack of energy? (*Please circle one number.*)
    (1) More than once a day
    (2) About once a day
    (3) More than once a week
    (4) About once a week
    (5) Rarely or never

8. Screening for Emotional Distress Mood Questionnaire

The following questionnaire (the Patient Health Questionnaire-9 [PHQ-9]) is designed to assess different aspects of your mood. Indicate your response using the categories on the right.

How often have you experienced the following problems in the past 2 weeks?

	Not at All	Several Days	More Than Half the Days	Nearly Every Day
1. Little interest or pleasure in doing things	0	1	2	3
2. Feeling down, depressed, or hopeless	0	1	2	3
3. Trouble falling asleep or staying asleep, or sleeping too much	0	1	2	3
4. Feeling tired or having little energy	0	1	2	3
5. Poor appetite or overeating	0	1	2	3
6. Feeling bad about yourself, or that you are a failure, or that you have let yourself or your family down	0	1	2	3
7. Trouble concentrating on things, such as reading the newspaper or watching television	0	1	2	3
8. Moving or speaking so slowly that other people could have noticed. Or the opposite—being so fidgety or restless that you have been moving around a lot more than usual	0	1	2	3
9. Thoughts that you would be better off dead or of hurting yourself in some way	0	1	2	3
Column Totals:		____ +	____ +	____
Add Column Totals Together:		____		

Scoring Instructions:

- Scores below 5 indicate no concern;
- Scores between 5 and 14 indicate some mild symptoms of difficulty with mood. You may be able to address these by seeking support from family and friends, beginning to work through a self-help book (see the Resources section on page 173 for suggestions), or making efforts to engage in more rewarding and pleasurable activities in your life;
- Scores of 15 or higher indicate symptoms of depression and likely warrant seeking help from a professional counselor and/or family physician.

Symptoms of Distress Questionnaire

The following questionnaire (Generalized Anxiety Disorder 7-Item [GAD-7] Scale) is designed to assess symptoms of distress. Using the categories on the right, indicate the most applicable answer for each item.

How often have you experienced the following problems in the past 2 weeks?

	Not at All	Several Days	More Than Half the Days	Nearly Every Day
1. Feeling nervous, anxious, or on edge	0	1	2	3
2. Not being able to stop or control worrying	0	1	2	3
3. Worrying too much about different things	0	1	2	3
4. Trouble relaxing	0	1	2	3
5. Being so restless that it is hard to sit still	0	1	2	3
6. Becoming easily annoyed or irritable	0	1	2	3
7. Feeling afraid, as if something awful might happen	0	1	2	3
Column Totals:		___ +	___ +	___
Add Totals Together:		___		

Scoring Instructions:

- Scores below 5 indicate no concern.
- Scores between 5 and 10 indicate some mild symptoms of difficulty with stress. You may be able to address these by seeking support from family and friends, beginning to work through a self-help book (see the Resources section on page 173 for suggestions), or practicing the relaxation exercises listed on pages 90 to 94.
- Scores over 10 indicate symptoms of anxiety and warrant seeking help from a professional counselor and/or family physician.

9. Beliefs Awareness Exercise

The instructions for this exercise can be found on pages 128 to 129.

Belief: _____

Challenge: _____

_____

_____

Belief: _____

Challenge: _____

_____

_____

Belief: _____

Challenge: _____

_____

_____

Belief: _____

Challenge: _____

_____

_____

GLOSSARY

ADT2—ADT where the patient takes both a luteinizing hormone-releasing hormone (LHRH) drug and also an antiandrogen drug. *See also* Androgen deprivation therapy, GnRH agonists and antagonists listed.

ADT3—ADT where the patient concurrently takes an LHRH drug, an antiandrogen drug, and a 5-alpha reductase inhibitor. *See also* Andrgen deprivation therapy.

Androgen—Any substance, such as testosterone or dihydrotestosterone, that promotes male characteristics (e.g., body hair growth).

Androgen deprivation therapy (ADT)—ADT, also known as hormone therapy, is a therapy designed to inhibit the body's production of androgens, testosterone in particular.

Antiandrogen—Drugs that prevent androgens from activating cells. Antiandrogens do this by competing with natural androgens for the appropriate receptors on the cells and blocking those receptors so that natural androgens cannot activate them. *See also* Androgen.

Body mass index (BMI)—A measure of whether a person is underweight, overweight, or obese, calculated from a person's weight and height.

Bone mineral density (BMD)—A measure of the amount of mineral in bone, which gives it its strength. Mild loss of BMD is called osteopenia and more serious loss is called osteoporosis. A person with osteoporosis is at increased risk of breaking a bone should he or she fall.

Brachytherapy—Treatment with ionizing radiation, usually in the form of small radioactive seeds or pellets. The pellets are inserted into the target organ.

Cardiovascular—This refers to the heart and the vessels that carry blood to and from the heart.

Castration—Removal of the testicles by surgery or making them inactive by chemical means so they cannot produce sperm or testosterone. Chemical and surgical castrations are equally effective in lowering testosterone levels. *See also* Androgen deprivation therapy, Orchiectomy.

Castration-resistant prostate cancer (CRPC)—Prostate cancer that cannot be controlled by ADT is said to be castration resistant. CRPC is indicated by a continuously rising prostate-specific antigen (PSA) despite ADT. If there are signs of metastases ("mets"), it is called **metastatic CRPC** (or **mCRPC**). *See also* Prostate-specific antigen.

Cognitive function—An intellectual process by which one becomes aware of, perceives, or comprehends ideas. It involves all aspects of perception, thinking, reasoning, and remembering.

Computed tomography (CT)—A form of diagnostic imaging that uses x-rays which creates cross-sectional and three-dimensional images of the body. Also referred to as a CAT scan.

Diethylstilbestrol (DES)—A synthetic (man-made) estrogen compound that was the first oral medication used for ADT, but was replaced by other drugs because it was associated with a high incidence of blood clot formation.

Dihydrotestosterone (DHT)—A natural androgen that is more potent than testosterone. It is produced in the body from testosterone by the enzyme 5-alpha reductase. *See also* Testosterone.

Dual-energy x-ray absorptiometry (DEXA or DXA)—A type of x-ray imaging used to measure bone mineral density.

Erectile dysfunction (ED)—Inability of a man to achieve and maintain an erection sufficient for satisfying penetrative sex.

Estradiol—The most potent naturally occurring estrogen found in both males and females. *See also* Estrogen.

Estrogen—Any of several steroid hormones that are secreted primarily by the ovaries and placenta in females. They promote the development of female secondary sex characteristics (e.g., breasts). In males, the primary estrogen is estradiol and it is normally made from testosterone by the enzyme aromatase. *See also* Hormones.

External beam radiation (EBRT)—A method of delivering high-energy x-rays to a patient's tumor. In contrast to brachytherapy, in EBRT the x-ray beams are generated outside the patient's body and targeted at the tumor.

5-alpha reductase—An enzyme that converts testosterone to a more potent androgen, dihydrotestosterone. Drugs that block the enzyme and thus the production of dihydrotestosterone are known as 5-alpha reductase inhibitors.

GnRH agonists and antagonists, also called LHRH agonists and antagonists— Two classes of synthetic (man-made) hormones that block, in different ways, a chemical signal from the **hypothalamus** in the brain to the **pituitary gland** at the base of the brain. This lack of chemical signal from the pituitary gland "tells" the testes to stop making **testosterone**. This shuts down testosterone production from the testicles. *See also* Hormones, LHRH agonists and antagonists.

Gynecomastia—A noncancerous increase in the size of the breasts in a male.

Hormones—Hormones are compounds in the body that are produced by endocrine glands and have specific target tissues in the body (e.g., breast, prostate). They activate or suppress activity in their target tissue. Hormones can be internally secreted or pharmacological products taken as drugs.

Hypothalamus—A region of the brain that coordinates the activity of the pituitary to control body temperature, sex hormone production, and several other bodily functions.

IU—International Units, an internationally accepted amount of a substance in pharmacology.

LHRH agonists and antagonists—These are alternative names for the two classes of synthetic hormones called GnRH agonists and antagonists, which stop the signal from the pituitary gland to the testicles to make testosterone. The **LHRH agonists** are the most common drugs used for ADT.

Mastalgia—Breast tenderness, sensitivity, and pain.

Meta-analysis—A statistical procedure that integrates the results of several independent studies to create a single, more robust estimate of an effect.

Metabolic syndrome—A condition associated with obesity, including elements such as glucose intolerance, insulin resistance, and raised blood pressure. It is associated with an increased risk of cardiovascular disease and diabetes.

Metastasis—The spread of cancer from an initial or primary site to a secondary site in the body. New sites are called **metastases ("mets")**. Cancer that has not metastasized is said to be **localized**. When prostate cancer has metastasized, the disease is said to be **systemic**. Most often prostate cancer metastasizes to the skeleton to form **bony mets**, but it can also spread to lymph nodes and other organs to form **soft tissue mets**.

Orchiectomy—Surgical removal of the testes. *See also* Castration.

Osteoporosis—A disorder in which the bones become increasingly porous, brittle, and subject to fracture, due to a loss of calcium and other mineral components. Osteoporotic fractures can lead to decreased height and skeletal deformities. Osteoporosis is common in older people, primarily postmenopausal women, but also is associated with androgen deprivation in men.

Glossary

Phosphodiesterase-5 inhibitors (PDE5i)—Drugs used to treat erectile dysfunction. These include the oral drugs Viagra®, Cialis®, Stendra®, and Levitra®. *See also* Erectile dysfunction.

Pituitary gland—A structure attached by a stalk to the base of the brain, which controls many of the hormonal pathways in the body.

Prostate-specific antigen (PSA)—A protein, produced by prostate cells, elevated levels of which may indicate the presence of prostate cancer or other prostatic disease. *See also* PSA test.

Prostatectomy—The surgical removal of part or all of the prostate gland.

PSA test—A blood test that measures the amount of PSA in the serum. *See also* Prostate-specific antigen.

Radiation therapy—Use of high-energy, penetrating waves or particles such as x-rays, gamma rays, proton beams, or neutron beams to destroy cancer cells or keep them from reproducing.

Sarcopenia—The loss of skeletal muscle mass that normally occurs with aging, but can be accelerated with ADT. When sarcopenia happens concurrently with weight gained as fat, the condition is called **sarcopenic obesity**.

SI—International System of Units, expressed as millimoles per litre (= mmol/L).

Testicles (Testes)—The male sex organs located in the scrotum, which produce sperm and the hormone testosterone.

Testosterone—The primary sex hormone in males, secreted by the testes, which stimulates the development of male sex organs, secondary sexual traits, and sperm. *See also* Androgen, Hormones.

RESOURCES

General

Finding Trustworthy Information Online

It is not difficult to find information about prostate cancer on the Internet. Indeed, a Google search on "prostate cancer" yields over 20 million hits! That is an impossible amount of information for anyone to plow through. So, one's searches need to be more specific. Suppose, though, that one searches on "prostate cancer" plus "androgen deprivation therapy." That still yields over 300,000 hits. Three strings of words entered together (with the quotes, which help find specific phrases)—"prostate cancer," "side effects," and "hormonal therapy"—cuts the number in half, but this is still too many sites.

So how does one decide what is worth looking at? What is reliable, and what is not?

It helps to understand the meaning of top-level domain names. These are indicated by the last three letters in a website's address. The common ones to be aware of are .edu, .gov, .org, and .com. ".edu" sites typically refer to academic organizations; that is, colleges and universities. ".gov" addresses are primarily for U.S. governmental agencies. ".org" historically meant noncommercial organization and ".com" designated a business, but those two categories are no longer well separated. In fact, the *www.LIFEonADT.com* site is primarily educational and not commercial. Generally though, the addresses with the most reliable information are those whose addresses end with the extensions of .gov, .edu, and, then .org.

Trustworthy sites are not necessarily embellished with music, animation, and videos. Sites with those fancy features are often commercial operations that aim to promote a product. Reliable sites clearly indicate who owns them.

If a site promotes a specific product for cancer treatment, it is wise to scroll to the bottom and look for small-print disclaimers. The owners of the site often display those disclaimers to acknowledge the limitations of their product. So, for example, the site might suggest that some herbal product is a "better way to fight cancer," but then have a disclaimer saying that such statements are not meant to endorse the product but instead for "educational purposes." The disclaimer is an effort to keep the owners out of legal trouble when the product has not been shown with solid, scientific research to be beneficial. It is better then to trust those disclaimers than the text that came before them.

Although there are exceptions to the following principles, websites with an extensive list of personal testimonials endorsing a particular cancer treatment or product should be viewed critically. Such testimonials are usually biased, presenting a one-sided, typically positive, view of a product. As a general rule, competent and responsible websites do not rely on testimonials to justify the materials or information they offer.

In an analysis of otherwise reliable websites for information on androgen deprivation therapy (ADT), many websites owned by major nonprofit, cancer-dedicated organizations were not up-to-date, even though they had a time stamp stating when they had last been updated. One website did stand out as having comprehensive current information: www.USTOO.org.

Another highly regarded and reliable site is the National Comprehensive Cancer Network (https://www.nccn.org/patients/default.aspx). The NCCN provides a free, online, comprehensive book about prostate cancer, which is regularly updated by their panel of expert oncologists and urologists (To access the book, go to: https://www.nccn.org/patients/guidelines/prostate/files/assets/basic-html/page-1.html#).

The LIFEonADT.com website

LIFEonADT.com is a website dedicated to the educational program associated with this book. The site should not be considered a definitive source for up-to-date information on ADT. The volume of medical information coming out weekly related to ADT is just too much for that site to assemble and summarize. One can though use "Google alerts" to get daily alerts on the topics of interest, such as ADT. To sign up for this service, go to www.google.com/alerts.

LIFEonADT.com Video Series: This site provides a link to videos we created that are associated with chapters in this book. The videos are posted on an external server and can be viewed there if you click on the thumbnail image for each video at LIFEonADT.com. You will then be prompted to enter a password. That can be obtained by a one-line email request to lifeonADT@gmail.com for the password.

Among the videos are a series related to the activities that you find at the end of the introduction and the following chapters in the book. These include instructional videos on

- Using the "Values Clarification Activity"
- Using the "Questions for Discussion"
- Completing an "Action Plan"
- Filling in a "Pros/Cons Table"

Additional videos include comments from patients and partners about their experience with ADT and its side effects. Sometimes people find it helpful to hear about other patients' experiences in addition to reading about the side effect management options that are the focus of this book. These videos provide personal perspectives on ADT and complement the information covered in the previous chapters.

Physical Side Effects

LIFEonADT.com Patient Video Series relevant topics:

- ADT-related changes
- Adjusting to physical changes from ADT
- Why learning about ADT is important
- Being proactive is important
- Dealing with hot flashes

Gynecomastia—Garments and compression shirts:

- www.underarmour.com
- www.amazon.com (search gynecomastia)
- www.underworks.com/microfiber-compression-tank

Healthy Lifestyle Resources

Physical activity, stress reduction, and nutrition website for prostate cancer patients:
lifestyle.truenth.ca

Exercise

Dr. Mike Evans Video Lecture: 23½ Hours:
    www.youtube.com/watch?v=aUaInS6HIGo

LIFEonADT.com Patient Video Series relevant topics:

- Dealing with fatigue and making adjustments
- Staying physically active
- Exercise combats fatigue
- Learning about ADT leads to a healthier lifestyle

Diet and Nutrition

Dr. Mike Evans Video Lecture: What Is the Best Diet? Healthy Eating 101:
 www.youtube.com/watch?v=fqhYBTg73fw

Prostate Cancer, Nutrition, and Dietary Supplements:
 www.cancer.gov/about-cancer/treatment/cam/patient/prostate-supplements-pdq

Canada Food Guide 2017:
 www.canada.ca/content/dam/hc-sc/migration/hc-sc/fn-an/alt_formats/hpfb-dgpsa/pdf/food-guide-aliment/print_eatwell_bienmang-eng.pdf

American Dietary Guidelines:
 health.gov/dietaryguidelines/2015/guidelines/introduction/dietary-guidelines-for-americans/

Canadian Guidelines for Body Weight Classification in Adults:
 www.canada.ca/en/health-canada/services/food-nutrition/healthy-eating/healthy-weights/canadian-guidelines-body-weight-classification-adults/questions-answers-public.html

Dietary Intake References

 Canada: www.hc-sc.gc.ca/fn-an/food-guide-aliment/index-eng.php
 United States: fnic.nal.usda.gov/dietary-guidance/dietary-reference-intakes

Psychological Well-Being

Katz, A. (2012). *Prostate cancer and the man you love: Supporting and caring for your partner*. Lanham, MD: Rowman & Littlefield.

LIFEonADT.com Patient Video Series relevant topics:

- Emotional changes due to ADT
- Dealing with increased emotional expression
- Getting psychological counseling
- Being single, getting support, and coping with ADT changes

Mindfulness Meditation Resources

Audio Recording
 Body Scan Meditation—Led by Jon Kabat-Zinn: youtu.be/_DTmGtznab4
Books
Full Catastrophe Living by Jon Kabat-Zinn (2013). This book provides a thorough overview of mindfulness and its application to health and illness.

Mindfulness-Based Cancer Recovery: A Step-by-Step MBSR Approach to Help You Cope With Treatment and Reclaim Your Life by Linda Carlson and Michael Speca (2011). This book covers an 8-week program that involves theory and practice designed specifically for cancer patients and their support persons.

Distress, Relaxation, and Coping Books

The Anxiety and Phobia Workbook by Edmund J. Bourne (2015). This workbook is an excellent step-by-step self-help program based on cognitive behavioral therapy that is highly effective in the treatment of anxiety disorders.

Feeling Good, the New Mood Therapy by David Burns (2008). This book presents cognitive behavioral therapy self-help strategies to help with depression.

Sexuality and Intimacy

Prostate Cancer UK—Sex & Prostate Cancer: Martin's Story: youtu.be/AV0yZIiWTng

LIFEonADT.com Patient Video Series relevant topics:

- Adjusting to the loss of spontaneous sex
- Changed view on sex
- Staying sexual
- Working with reduced sexual interest
- Staying connected in ways other than sex
- Remaining close without being sexual
- Being OK without sex
- Sexual tips
- Challenges in dating

Support Services, Both Face-to-Face and Online

The Global Prostate Cancer Alliance (prostatecanceralliance.org) has direct links to most of the major prostate cancer patient organizations worldwide. These can be accessed by clicking on their logos posted at prostatecanceralliance.org/current-members/. Many of the groups listed there provide online forums, discussion boards, Internet chat groups, and some also sponsor face-to-face meetings for both patients and partners.

Some of the more prominent organizations in North America that provide support services include the following:

- Us TOO—Us TOO sponsors face-to-face support groups in the United States. See www.ustoo.org/Home. Us TOO also has online discussion boards accessible at www.ustoo.inspire.com;

- The Prostate Net—They offer support to patients accessible at support@prostatenet.org;
- Malecare—Malecare.org has a variety of support services both of the face-to-face format and online. Its online discussion boards are managed by healthunlocked.com and their many chat groups. The one that has the most discussion about ADT is accessible at healthunlocked.com/advanced-prostate-cancer;
- Prostate Cancer International (PCaI)—The "New" Prostate Cancer InfoLink Social Network is a service of PCaI and is closely associated with the regular research news updates it provides through its subscription service at The "New" Prostate Cancer InfoLink. PCaI has many chat groups, some more active than others. The group most relevant to ADT is accessible at prostatecancerinfolink.ning.com/group/hormonesuppression. The "New" Prostate Cancer InfoLink also offers some well-organized lists of prostate cancer advocacy and support organizations around the world. Although its lists are not completely up-to-date—organizations come and go—they are impressively comprehensive and well annotated;

Information for major U.S.-based prostate cancer websites and organizations can be found at prostatecancerinfolink.net/tips-tools/us-based-prostate-cancer-web-sites.
For organizations outside the United States, go to prostatecancerinfolink.net/tips-tools/ex-us-prostate-cancer-web-sites.

- Prostate Cancer Canada has its network, which is a collection of face-to-face groups across Canada. Information on the network and other support services that Prostate Cancer Canada provides is accessible at www.prostatecancer.ca/Supporting-You/Services/Support-Groups;
- The Prostate Cancer Research Institute is another organization that has a comprehensive list of local support groups across the organized by state. It can be found at: https://pcri.org/supportgroups
- Finally, there are resources available specifically for the partners of patients. A lead to such resources can be found at www.hisprostatecancer.com/prostate-cancer-support-groups.html. An active women's only discussion board run by the Ladies Prostate Forum is accessible at www.ladies-prostate-forum.org/ladies

For Gay Men With Prostate Cancer

Support groups

- MaleCare.com
- healthunlocked.com/prostate-cancer-gay-men/posts

- www.facebook.com/GayProstateCancerSupport
- www.prostate.org.au/support/find-a-support-group/sydney-shine-a-light-support-group-for-gay-and-bisexual-men (Australia)
- prostate.org.nz/rainbow-blue (New Zealand)

General Information for Gay and Bisexual Prostate Cancer Patients

- prostatecancer.ca/Prostate-Cancer/Care-and-Support-Post-Treatment/Gay-and-Bisexual-Men-Prostate-Cancer
- www.prostate.org.au/awareness/for-recently-diagnosed-men-and-their-families/gay-and-bisexual-men
- prostatecanceruk.org/prostate-information/living-with-prostate-cancer/gay-and-bisexual-men
- malecare.org/gay-prostate-cancer-and-doctors
- www.cancercare.org/support_groups/105-cancer_i_care_i_sage_gay_male_cancer_survivors_support_group

Book

Gay and bisexual men living with prostate cancer: From diagnosis to recovery, edited by Perz and Simon Rosser (2018).

Comparing Different Treatments

Prostate Cancer Free Foundation (PCFF)—This foundation is a relatively new organization with a unique mission. As such, we list it here in its own category. PCFF sponsors the Prostate Cancer Results Study Group, which reviews the medical literature for treatment-related articles. The Study Group has developed analytical tools to graphically summarize its findings in a way that can help patients visualize the effectiveness of various treatments. Its charts and graphs, which are updated every 6 months, take into consideration whether patients are considered at low, medium, or high risk of advanced disease. A link to their findings is https://prostatecancerfree.org/prostate-cancer-treatments.

BIBLIOGRAPHY

The following list of journal articles are representative of the literature accessed during the development of this book. This is not a definitive list of the papers reviewed. Many of the papers listed under one topic fit equally well under other topics. We have not, however, repeated the citations to avoid inflating the overall length of the list.

The papers selected for listing here are relatively recent (i.e., mostly published in the last few years) and most are Open Access (i.e., accessible online for free). If you use the PubMed search engine (www.pubmed.com), you can read the abstracts of the papers. If you then click on the side where it says "open access" or "free full text," you should be able to retrieve the full article.

Introduction to Androgen Deprivation Therapy (ADT)

Dell'Oglio, P., Bishr, M., Boehm, K., Trudeau, V., Larcher, A., Tian, Z., . . . Karakiewicz, P. I. (2017). Survival outcomes in octogenarian and nonagenarian patients treated with first-line androgen deprivation therapy for organ-confined prostate cancer. *European Urology Focus*. Advance online publication. doi:10.1016/j.euf.2017.01.017.

Hussain, M., Tangen, C. M., Berry, D. L., Higano, C. S., Crawford, E. D., Liu, G., . . . Thompson, I. M., Jr. (2013). Intermittent versus continuous androgen deprivation in prostate cancer. *New England Journal of Medicine*, *368*(14), 1314–1325. doi:10.1056/NEJMoa1212299

Hussain, M., Tangen, C., Higano, C., Vogelzang, N., & Thompson, I. (2016). Evaluating intermittent androgen-deprivation therapy phase III clinical trials: The devil is in the details. *Journal of Clinical Oncology*, *34*(3), 280–285. doi:10.1200/JCO.2015.62.8065

Lin, Y. H., Chen, C. L., Hou, C. P., Chang, P. L., & Tsui, K. H. (2011). A comparison of androgen deprivation therapy versus surgical castration for patients with advanced prostatic carcinoma. *Acta Pharmacologica Sinica, 32*(4), 537–542. doi:10.1038/aps.2010.236

Rot, I., Wassersug, R. J., & Walker, L. M. (2016). What do urologists think patients need to know when starting on androgen deprivation therapy? The perspective from Canada versus countries with lower gross domestic product. *Translational Andrology and Urology, 5*(2), 235–247. doi:10.21037/tau.2016.03.06

Spratt, D. E., Dess, R. T., Zumsteg, Z. S., Lin, D. W., Tran, P. T., Morgan, T. M., . . . Feng, F. Y. (2018). A systematic review and framework for the use of hormone therapy with salvage radiation therapy for recurrent prostate cancer. *European Urology, 73*(2), 156–165. doi:10.1016/j.eururo.2017.06.027

Taguchi, S., Fukuhara, H., Morikawa, T., Matsumoto, A., Miyazaki, H., Nakagawa, T., . . . Homma, Y. (2016). Cessation of long-term adjuvant androgen deprivation therapy after radical prostatectomy: Is it feasible? *Japanese Journal of Clinical Oncology, 46*(12), 1143–1147. doi:10.1093/jjco/hyw136

Walker, L. M., Tran, S., Wassersug, R. J., Thomas, B., & Robinson, J. W. (2013). Patients and partners lack knowledge of androgen deprivation therapy side effects. *Urologic Oncology, 31*(7), 1098–1105. doi: 10.1016/j.urolonc.2011.12.015

Warde, P., Mason, M., Ding, K., Kirkbride, P., Brundage, M., Cowan, R., . . . Parulekar, W. (2011). Combined androgen deprivation therapy and radiation therapy for locally advanced prostate cancer: A randomised, phase 3 trial. *Lancet, 378*(9809), 2104–2111. doi:10.1016/S0140-6736(11)61095-7

Yano, A., Kagawa, M., Takeshita, H., Okada, Y., Morozumi, M., & Kawakami, S. (2017). Improved survival of men with metastatic prostate cancer treated with androgen deprivation therapy plus radiotherapy to the prostate. *International Journal of Urology, 24*(12), 863–865. doi:10.1111/iju.13479

Understanding the Physical Side Effects of ADT

Ahmadi, H., & Daneshmand, S. (2013). Androgen deprivation therapy: Evidence-based management of side effects. *BJU International, 111*(4), 543–548. doi:10.1111/j.1464-410X.2012.11774.x

Allan, C., Collins, V. R., Frydenberg, M., McLachlan, R. I., & Matthiesson, K. L. (2014). Androgen deprivation therapy complications. *Endocrine-Related Cancer, 21*(4), T119–T129. doi.org/10.1530/ERC-13-0467

Elliott, S., Latini, D. M., Walker, L. M., Wassersug, R., & Robinson, J. W. (2010). Androgen deprivation therapy for prostate cancer: Recommendations to improve patient and partner quality of life. *Journal of Sexual Medicine, 7*(9), 2996–3010. doi:10.1111/j.1743-6109.2010.01902.x

Nguyen, P. L., Alibhai, S. M., Basaria, S., D'Amico, A. V., Kantoff, P. W., Keating, N. L., . . . Smith, M. R. (2015). Adverse effects of androgen deprivation therapy and strategies to mitigate them. *European Urology*, 67(5), 825–836. doi: 10.1016/j.eururo.2014.07.010

Saylor, P. J., & Smith, M. R. (2010). Adverse effects of androgen deprivation therapy: Defining the problem and promoting health among men with prostate cancer. *Journal of the National Comprehensive Cancer Network*, 8(2), 211–223. doi:10.6004/jnccn.2010.0014

Cardiovascular and Diabetic Risk

Bosco, C., Crawley, D., Adolfsson, J., Rudman, S., & Van Hemelrijck, M. (2015). Quantifying the evidence for the risk of metabolic syndrome and its components following androgen deprivation therapy for prostate cancer: A meta-analysis. *PLOS ONE*, 10(3), e0117344. doi:10.1371/journal.pone.0117344

Crawley, D., Garmo, H., Rudman, S., Stattin, P., Haggstrom, C., Zethelius, B., . . . Van Hemelrijck, M. (2016). Association between duration and type of androgen deprivation therapy and risk of diabetes in men with prostate cancer. *International Journal of Cancer*, 139(12), 2698–2704. doi:10.1002/ijc.30403

Gacci, M., Russo, G. I., De Nunzio, C., Sebastianelli, A., Salvi, M., Vignozzi, L., . . . Serni, S. (2017). Meta-analysis of metabolic syndrome and prostate cancer. *Prostate Cancer and Prostatic Diseases*, 20(2), 146–155. doi:10.1038/pcan.2017.1

Gilbert, S. E., Tew, G. A., Fairhurst, C., Bourke, L., Saxton, J. M., Winter, E. M., & Rosario, D. J. (2016). Effects of a lifestyle intervention on endothelial function in men on long-term androgen deprivation therapy for prostate cancer. *British Journal of Cancer*, 114(4), 401–408. doi:10.1038/bjc.2015.479

Karzai, F. H., Madan, R. A., & Dahut, W. L. (2016). Metabolic syndrome in prostate cancer: Impact on risk and outcomes. *Future Oncology*, 12(16), 1947–1955. doi:10.2217/fon-2016-0061

Keating, N. L., Liu, P. H., O'Malley, A. J., Freedland, S. J., & Smith, M. R. (2014). Androgen-deprivation therapy and diabetes control among diabetic men with prostate cancer. *European Urology*, 65(4), 816–824. doi:10.1016/j.eururo.2013.02.023

Kiwata, J. L., Dorff, T. B., Schroeder, E. T., Gross, M. E., & Dieli-Conwright, C. M. (2016). A review of clinical effects associated with metabolic syndrome and exercise in prostate cancer patients. *Prostate Cancer and Prostatic Diseases*, 19(4), 323–332. doi:10.1038/pcan.2016.25

Mitsuzuka, K., & Arai, Y. (2017). Metabolic changes in patients with prostate cancer during androgen deprivation therapy. *International Journal of Urology*, 25(1), 45–53. doi:10.1111/iju.13473

Rudman, S. M., Gray, K. P., Batista, J. L., Pitt, M. J., Giovannucci, E. L., Harper, P. G., . . . Sweeney, C. J. (2016). Risk of prostate cancer specific death in men with baseline metabolic aberrations treated with androgen deprivation therapy for biochemical recurrence. *BJU International*, *118*(6), 919–926. doi:10.1111/bju.13428

Spratt, D. E., Zhang, C., Zumsteg, Z. S., Pei, X., Zhang, Z., & Zelefsky, M. J. (2013). Metformin and prostate cancer: Reduced development of castration-resistant disease and prostate cancer mortality. *European Urology*, *63*(4), 709–716. doi:10.1016/j.eururo.2012.12.004

Thomsen, F. B., Sandin, F., Garmo, H., Lissbrant, I. F., Ahlgren, G., Van Hemelrijck, M., . . . Stattin, P. (2017). Gonadotropin-releasing hormone agonists, orchiectomy, and risk of cardiovascular disease: Semi-ecologic, nationwide, population-based study. *European Urology*, *72*(6), 920–928. doi:10.1016/j.eururo.2017.06.036

Tzortzis, V., Samarinas, M., Zachos, I., Oeconomou, A., Pisters, L. L., & Bargiota, A. (2017). Adverse effects of androgen deprivation therapy in patients with prostate cancer: Focus on metabolic complications. *Hormones*, *16*(2), 115–123. doi:10.14310/horm.2002.1727

Whitburn, J., Edwards, C. M., & Sooriakumaran, P. (2017). Metformin and prostate cancer: A new role for an old drug. *Current Urology Reports*, *18*(6), 46. doi:10.1007/s11934-017-0693-8

Zareba, P., Duivenvoorden, W., Leong, D. P., & Pinthus, J. H. (2016). Androgen deprivation therapy and cardiovascular disease: What is the linking mechanism? *Therapeutic Advances in Urology*, *8*(2), 118–129. doi:10.1177/1756287215617872

Hot Flashes

Ahmadi, H., & Daneshmand, S. (2014). Androgen deprivation therapy for prostate cancer: Long-term safety and patient outcomes. *Patient Related Outcome Measures*, *5*, 63–70. doi:10.2147/PROM.S52788

Challapalli, A., Edwards, S. M., Abel, P., & Mangar, S. A. (2018). Evaluating the prevalence and predictive factors of vasomotor and psychological symptoms in prostate cancer patients receiving hormonal therapy: Results from a single institution experience. *Clinical and Translational Radiation Oncology*, *10*, 29–35. doi:10.1016/j.ctro.2018.03.002

Frisk, J. (2010). Managing hot flushes in men after prostate cancer—A systematic review. *Maturitas*, *65*(1), 15–22. doi:10.1016/j.maturitas.2009.10.017

Hunter, M. S., & Stefanopoulou, E. (2016). Vasomotor symptoms in prostate cancer survivors undergoing androgen deprivation therapy. *Climacteric*, *19*(1), 91–97. doi:10.3109/13697137.2015.1125460

Johns, C., Seav, S. M., Dominick, S. A., Gorman, J. R., Li, H., Natarajan, L., . . . Irene Su, H. (2016). Informing hot flash treatment decisions for breast cancer survivors: A systematic review of randomized trials comparing active interventions. *Breast Cancer Research and Treatment*, *156*(3), 415–426. doi:10.1007/s10549-016-3765-4

Phillips, I., Shah, S. I., Duong, T., Abel, P., & Langley, R. E. (2014). Androgen deprivation therapy and the re-emergence of parenteral estrogen in prostate cancer. *Oncology & Hematology Review*, *10*(1), 42–47. doi:10.17925/OHR.2014.10.1.42

Bone Health

Beebe-Dimmer, J. L., Cetin, K., Shahinian, V., Morgenstern, H., Yee, C., Schwartz, K. L., & Acquavella, J. (2012). Timing of androgen deprivation therapy use and fracture risk among elderly men with prostate cancer in the United States. *Pharmacoepidemiology and Drug Safety*, *21*(1), 70–78. doi:10.1002/pds.2258

Bolam, K. A., Galvão, D. A., Spry, N., Newton, R. U., & Taaffe, D. R. (2012). AST-induced bone loss in men with prostate cancer: Exercise as a potential countermeasure. *Prostate Cancer and Prostatic Diseases*, *15*(4), 329–338. doi:10.1038/pcan.2012.22

Canadian Agency for Drugs and Technologies in Health. (2016). Denosumab versus zoledronic acid for men with osteoporosis: A review of clinical effectiveness and guidelines. *CADTH Rapid Response Reports*. Ottawa, ON, Canada: Author. Retrieved from https://www.ncbi.nlm.nih.gov/pubmedhealth/PMH0090372

Cianferotti, L., Bertoldo, F., Carini, M., Kanis, J. A., Lapini, A., Longo, N., . . . Brandi, M. L. (2017). The prevention of fragility fractures in patients with non-metastatic prostate cancer: A position statement by the International Osteoporosis Foundation. *Oncotarget*, *8*(43), 75646–75663. doi:10.18632/oncotarget.17980

Kim, S. H., Joung, J. Y., Kim, S., Rha, K. H., Kim, H. G., Kwak, C., . . . Kim, C. S. (2017). Comparison of bone mineral loss by combined androgen block agonist versus GnRH in patients with prostate cancer: A 12-month prospective observational study. *Scientific Reports*, *7*, 39562. doi:10.1038/srep39562

Kirk, P. S., Borza, T., Shahinian, V. B., Caram, M. E. V., Makarov, D. V., Shelton, J. B., . . . Skolarus, T. A. (2018). The implications of baseline bone-health assessment at initiation of androgen-deprivation therapy for prostate cancer. *BJU International*, *121*(4), 558–564. doi:10.1111/bju.14075

Macherey, S., Monsef, I., Jahn, F., Jordan, K., Yuen, K. K., Heidenreich, A., & Skoetz, N. (2017). Bisphosphonates for advanced prostate cancer. *Cochrane Database of Systematic Reviews*, *12*, CD006250. doi:10.1002/14651858.CD006250.pub2

Weight Gain

Braunstein, L. Z., Chen, M. H., Loffredo, M., Kantoff, P. W., & D'Amico, A. V. (2014). Obesity and the odds of weight gain following androgen deprivation therapy for prostate cancer. *Prostate Cancer, 2014,* 230812. doi:10.1155/2014/230812

Hojan, K., Kwiatkowska-Borowczyk, E., Leporowska, E., & Milecki, P. (2017). Inflammation, cardiometabolic markers, and functional changes in men with prostate cancer. A randomized controlled trial of a 12-month exercise program. *Polish Archives of Internal Medicine, 127*(1), 25–35. doi:10.20452/pamw.3888

Kim, H. S., Moreira, D. M., Smith, M. R., Presti, J. C., Jr, Aronson W. J., Terris, M. K., . . . Freedland, S. J. (2011). A natural history of weight change in men with prostate cancer on androgen-deprivation therapy (ADT): Results from the Shared Equal Access Regional Cancer Hospital (SEARCH) database. *BJU International, 107*(6), 924–928. doi:10.1111/j.1464-410X.2010.09679.x

Kirk, P. S., Borza, T., Shahinian, V. B., Caram, M. E. V., Makarov, D. V., Shelton, J. B., . . . Skolarus, T. A. (2018). The implications of baseline bone-health assessment at initiation of androgen-deprivation therapy for prostate cancer. *BJU International, 121(4), 558–564.* doi:10.1111/bju.14075

Fatigue

Engl, T., Drescher, D., Bickeboller, R., & Grabhorn, R. (2017). Fatigue, depression, and quality of life in patients with prostatic diseases. *Central European Journal of Urology, 70*(1), 44–47. doi:10.5173/ceju.2017.940

Nelson, A. M., Gonzalez, B. D., Jim, H. S., Cessna, J. M., Sutton, S. K., Small, B. J., . . . Jacobsen, P. B. (2016). Characteristics and predictors of fatigue among men receiving androgen deprivation therapy for prostate cancer: A controlled comparison. *Supportive Care in Cancer, 24*(10), 4159–4166. doi:10.1007/s00520-016-3241-z

Owen, P. J., Daly, R. M., Livingston, P. M., & Fraser, S. F. (2017). Lifestyle guidelines for managing adverse effects on bone health and body composition in men treated with androgen deprivation therapy for prostate cancer: An update. *Prostate Cancer and Prostatic Diseases, 20*(2), 137–145. doi:10.1038/pcan.2016.69

Exercise Recommendations for Patients on ADT

Fletcher, G. F., Ades, P. A., Kligfield, P., Arena, R., Balady, G. J., Bittner, V. A., . . . Council on Epidemiology and Prevention. (2013). Exercise standards for testing and training: A scientific statement from the American Heart Association. *Circulation, 128*(8), 873–934. doi:10.1038/pcan.2016.69

Gaskin, C. J., Fraser, S. F., Owen, P. J., Craike, M., Orellana, L., & Livingston, P. M. (2016). Fitness outcomes from a randomised controlled trial of exercise training for men with prostate cancer: The ENGAGE study. *Journal of Cancer Survivorship, 10*(6), 972–980. doi:10.1007/s11764-016-0543-6

Gonzalez, B. D., Jim, H. S., Small, B. J., Sutton, S. K., Fishman, M. N., Zachariah, B., . . . Jacobsen, P. B. (2016). Changes in physical functioning and muscle strength in men receiving androgen deprivation therapy for prostate cancer: A controlled comparison. *Supportive Care in Cancer, 24*(5), 2201–2207. doi:10.1007/s00520-015-3016-y

Moyad, M. A., Newton, R. U., Tunn, U. W., & Gruca, D. (2016). Integrating diet and exercise into care of prostate cancer patients on androgen deprivation therapy. *Research and Reports in Urology, 8*, 133–143. doi:10.2147/RRU.S107852

Taaffe, D. R., Newton, R. U., Spry, N., Joseph, D., Chambers, S. K., Gardiner, R. A., . . . Galvao, D. A. (2017). Effects of different exercise modalities on fatigue in prostate cancer patients undergoing androgen deprivation therapy: A year-long randomised controlled trial. *European Urology, 72*(2), 293–299. doi:10.1016/j.eururo.2017.02.019

Teleni, L., Chan, R. J., Chan, A., Isenring, E. A., Vela, I., Inder, W., & McCarthy, A. L. (2016). Exercise improves quality of life in ADT-treated prostate cancer: Systematic review of RCTs. *Endocrine-Related Cancer, 23*(2), 101–112. doi:10.1530/ERC-15-0456

Yunfeng, G., Weiyang, H., Xueyang, H., Yilong, H., & Xin, G. (2017). Exercise overcome adverse effects among prostate cancer patients receiving androgen deprivation therapy: An update meta-analysis. *Medicine, 96*(27), e7368. doi:10.1097/MD.0000000000007368

Healthy Eating and ADT

Anderson, J. J., Kruszka, B., Delaney, J. A., He, K., Burke, G. L., Alonso, A., . . . Michos, E. D. (2016). Calcium intake from diet and supplements and the risk of coronary artery calcification and its progression among older adults: 10-year follow-up of the multi-ethnic study of atherosclerosis (MESA). *Journal of the American Heart Association, 5*(10), e003815. doi:10.1161/JAHA.116.003815

Brasky, T. M., Darke, A. K., Song, X., Tangen, C. M., Goodman, P. J., Thompson, I. M., . . . Kristal, A. R. (2013). Plasma phospholipid fatty acids and prostate cancer risk in the SELECT trial. *Journal of the National Cancer Institute, 105*(15), 1015–1016. doi:10.1093/jnci/djt174.

Hardin, J., Cheng, I., & Witte, J. S. (2011). Impact of consumption of vegetable, fruit, grain, and high glycemic index foods on aggressive prostate cancer risk. *Nutrition and Cancer, 63*(6), 860–872. doi:10.1080/01635581.2011.582224

Harvard University School of Public Health. (2017). Calcium sources in food. Retrieved from https://www.hsph.harvard.edu/nutritionsource/calcium-sources

Health Canada. (2007). What is a food guide serving of meat and alternatives? Retrieved from https://www.canada.ca/en/health-canada/services/food-nutrition/canada-food-guide/choosing-foods/meat-alternatives/what-food-guide-serving-meat-alternatives.html

Hori, S., Butler, E., & McLoughlin, J. (2011). Prostate cancer and diet: Food for thought? *BJU International, 107*(9), 1348–1359. doi:10.1111/j.1464-410X.2010.09897.x.

National Cancer Institute. (2009). Calcium and cancer prevention. Retrieved from https://www.cancer.gov/about-cancer/causes-prevention/risk/diet/calcium-fact-sheet#q4

Nimptsch, K., Kenfield, S., Jensen, M. K., Stampfer, M. J., Franz, M., Sampson, L., ... Giovannucci, E. (2011). Dietary glycemic index, glycemic load, insulin index, fiber and whole-grain intake in relation to risk of prostate cancer. *Cancer Causes & Control, 22*(1), 51–61. doi:10.1007/s10552-010-9671-x

Office of Dietary Supplements. (2013). Dietary supplement fact sheet: Calcium. *National Institutes of Health.* Retrieved from https://ods.od.nih.gov/factsheets/Calcium-HealthProfessional

Waldman, T., Sarbaziha, R., Merz, C. N., & Shufelt, C. (2015). Calcium supplements and cardiovascular disease: A review. *American Journal of Lifestyle Medicine, 9*(4), 298–307. doi:10.1177/1559827613512593

Zhao, J. G., Zeng, X. T., Wang, J., & Liu, L. (2017). Association between calcium or vitamin D supplementation and fracture incidence in community-dwelling older adults: A systematic review and meta-analysis. *Journal of the American Medical Association, 318*(24), 2466–2482. doi:10.1001/jama.2017.19344

Effects on Mood and Emotional Well-Being

Dinh, K. T., Reznor, G., Muralidhar, V., Mahal, B. A., Nezolosky, M. D., Choueiri, T. K., ... Nguyen, P. L. (2016). Association of androgen deprivation therapy with depression in localized prostate cancer. *Journal of Clinical Oncology, 34*(16), 1905–1912. doi:10.1200/JCO.2015.64.1969

Dinh, K. T., Yang, D. D., Nead, K. T., Reznor, G., Trinh, Q. D., & Nguyen, P. L. (2017). Association between androgen deprivation therapy and anxiety among 78 000 patients with localized prostate cancer. *International Journal of Urology, 24*(10), 743–748. doi:10.1111/iju.13409

Gagliano-Juca, T., Travison, T. G., Nguyen, P. L., Kantoff, P. W., Taplin, M. E., Kibel, A. S., ... Basaria, S. (2018). Effects of androgen deprivation therapy on pain perception, quality of life, and depression in men with prostate cancer. *Journal of Pain and Symptom Management, 55*, 307–317. doi:10.1016/j.jpainsymman.2017.09.017

Kan, C., Silva, N., Golden, S. H., Rajala, U., Timonen, M., Stahl, D., & Ismail, K. (2013). A systematic review and meta-analysis of the association between depression and insulin resistance. *Diabetes Care*, 36(2), 480–489. doi:10.2337/dc12-1442

Pascoe, E. C., & Edvardsson, D. (2016). Which coping strategies can predict beneficial feelings associated with prostate cancer? *Journal of Clinical Nursing*, 25(17–18), 2569–2578. doi:10.1111/jocn.13300

Van Dam, D., Wassersug, R. J., & Hamilton, L. D. (2015). Androgen deprivation therapy's impact on the mood of prostate cancer patients as perceived by patients and the partners of patients. *Psychooncology*, 25(7), 848–856. doi:10.1002/pon.3932

Wikman, A., Wardle, J., & Steptoe, A. (2011). Quality of life and affective well-being in middle-aged and older people with chronic medical illnesses: A cross-sectional population based study. *PLOS ONE*, 6(4), e18952. doi:10.1371/journal.pone.0018952

Zhang, Z., Yang, L., Xie, D., Shi, H., Li, G., & Yu, D. (2017). Depressive symptoms are found to be potential adverse effects of androgen deprivation therapy in older prostate cancer patients: A 15-month prospective, observational study. *Psychooncology*, 26(12), 2238–2244. doi:10.1002/pon.4453

Effects on Cognition

Donovan, K. A., Walker, L. M., Wassersug, R. J., Thompson, L. M., & Robinson, J. W. (2015). Psychological effects of androgen-deprivation therapy on men with prostate cancer and their partners. *Cancer*, 121(24), 4286–4299. doi:10.1002/cncr.29672

Jamadar, R. J., Winters, M. J., & Maki, P. M. (2012). Cognitive changes associated with ADT: A review of the literature. *Asian Journal of Andrology*, 14(2), 232–238. doi:10.1038/aja.2011.107

Kao, L. T., Lin, H. C., Chung, S. D., & Huang, C. Y. (2016). No increased risk of dementia in patients receiving androgen deprivation therapy for prostate cancer: A 5-year follow-up study. *Asian Journal of Andrology*, 19(4), 414–417. doi:10.4103/1008-682X.179528

Kim, J. H., Lee, B., Han, D. H., Chung, K. J., Jeong, I. G., & Chung, B. I. (2017). Discrepancies on the association between androgen deprivation therapy for prostate cancer and subsequent dementia: Meta-analysis and meta-regression. *Oncotarget*, 8(42), 73087–73097. doi:10.18632/oncotarget.20391

Morote, J., Tabernero, A. J., Alvarez Ossorio, J. L., Ciria, J. P., Dominguez-Escrig, J. L., Vazquez, F., . . . Group, A. I. (2017). Cognitive function in patients with prostate cancer receiving luteinizing hormone-releasing hormone analogues: A prospective, observational, multicenter study. *International Journal of Radiation Oncology, Biology, Physics*, 98(3), 590–594. doi:10.1016/j.ijrobp.2017.02.219

Mundell, N. L., Daly, R. M., Macpherson, H., & Fraser, S. F. (2017). Cognitive decline in prostate cancer patients undergoing ADT. *Endocrine-Related Cancer*, 24(4), R145–R155. doi:10.1530/ERC-16-0493

Nead, K. T., Sinha, S., & Nguyen, P. L. (2017). Androgen deprivation therapy for prostate cancer and dementia risk: A systematic review and meta-analysis. *Prostate Cancer and Prostatic Diseases*, 20(3), 259–264. doi:10.1038/pcan.2017.10

Wu, L. M., Amidi, A., Tanenbaum, M. L., Winkel, G., Gordon, W. A., Hall, S. J., . . . Diefenbach, M. A. (2017). Computerized cognitive training in prostate cancer patients on androgen deprivation therapy: A pilot study. *Supportive Care in Cancer*. doi:10.1007/s00520-017-4026-8

Wu, L. M., Tanenbaum, M. L., Dijkers, M. P. J. M., Amidi, A., Hall, S. J., Penedo, F. J., & Diefenbach, M. A. (2016). Cognitive and neurobehavioral symptoms in patients with non-metastatic prostate cancer treated with androgen deprivation therapy or observation: A mixed methods study. *Social Science & Medicine*, 156, 80–89. doi:10.1016/j.socscimed.2016.03.016

Effects on Sexuality

Barbera, L., Zwaal, C., Elterman, D., McPherson, K., Wolfman, W., Katz, A., . . . Interventions to Address Sexual Problems in People With Cancer Guideline Development Group. (2017). Interventions to address sexual problems in people with cancer. *Current Oncology*, 24(3), 192–200. doi:10.3747/co.24.3583

Gay, H. A., Sanda, M. G., Liu, J., Wu, N., Hamstra, D. A., Wei, J. T., . . . Michalski, J. M. (2017). External beam radiation therapy or brachytherapy with or without short-course neoadjuvant androgen deprivation therapy: Results of a multicenter, prospective study of quality of life. *International Journal of Radiation Oncology, Biology, Physics*, 98(2), 304–317. doi:10.1016/j.ijrobp.2017.02.019

Palmer-Hague, J. L., Tsang, V., Skead, C., Wassersug, R. J., Nasiopoulos, E., & Kingstone, A. (2017). Androgen deprivation alters attention to sexually provocative visual stimuli in elderly men. *Sexual Medicine*, 5(4), e245–e254. doi:10.1016/j.esxm.2017.10.001

Walker, L. M., Hampton, A. J., Wassersug, R. J., Thomas, B. C., & Robinson, J. W. (2013). Androgen deprivation therapy and maintenance of intimacy: A randomized controlled pilot study of an educational intervention for patients and their partners. *Contemporary Clinical Trials*, 34(2), 227–231. doi:10.1016/j.cct.2012.11.007

Walker, L. M., Wassersug, R. J., & Robinson, J. W. (2015). Psychosocial perspectives on sexual recovery after prostate cancer treatment. *Nature Reviews. Urology*, 12(3), 167–176. doi:10.1038/nrurol.2015.29

Wassersug, R., & Wibowo, E. (2017). Non-pharmacological and non-surgical strategies to promote sexual recovery for men with erectile dysfunction. *Translational Andrology and Urology, 6*(Suppl. 5), S776–S794. doi:10.21037/tau.2017.04.09

Effects on Intimate Relationships

Hamilton, L. D., Van Dam, D., & Wassersug, R. J. (2015). The perspective of prostate cancer patients and patients' partners on the psychological burden of androgen deprivation and the dyadic adjustment of prostate cancer couples. *Psychooncology, 25*(7), 823–831. doi:10.1002/pon.3930

Navon, L., & Morag, A. (2003). Advanced prostate cancer patients' relationships with their spouses following hormonal therapy. *European Journal of Oncology Nursing, 7*(2), 73-80. doi:10.1016/S1462-3889(03)00022-X

Walker, L. M., & Robinson, J. W. (2010). The unique needs of couples experiencing androgen deprivation therapy for prostate cancer. *Journal of Sex & Marital Therapy, 36*(2), 154–165. doi:10.1080/00926230903554552

Walker, L. M., & Robinson, J. W. (2011). A description of heterosexual couples' sexual adjustment to androgen deprivation therapy for prostate cancer. *Psychooncology, 20*(8), 880–888. doi:10.1002/pon.1794

Wassersug, R. J. (2016). Maintaining intimacy for prostate cancer patients on androgen deprivation therapy. *Current Opinion in Supportive and Palliative Care, 10*(1), 55–65. doi:10.1097/SPC.0000000000000190

Newer ADT Agents

Devlin, N., Herdman, M., Pavesi, M., Phung Naidoo, S., Beer, T. M., Tombal, B., . . . Holmstrom, S. (2017). Health-related quality of life effects of enzalutamide in patients with metastatic castration-resistant prostate cancer: An in-depth post hoc analysis of EQ-5D data from the PREVAIL trial. *Health and Quality of Life Outcomes, 15*(1), 130. doi:10.1186/s12955-017-0704-y.

El-Amm, J., Nassabein, R., & Aragon-Ching, J. B. (2017). Impact of abiraterone on patient-related outcomes in metastatic castration-resistant prostate cancer: Current perspectives. *Cancer Management and Research, 2017*(9), 299–306. doi:10.2147/CMAR.S139305

Heidenreich, A., Chowdhury, S., Klotz, L., Siemens, D. R., Villers, A., Ivanescu, C., . . . Shore, N. D. (2017). Impact of enzalutamide compared with bicalutamide on quality of life in men with metastatic castration-resistant prostate cancer: Additional analyses from the TERRAIN randomised clinical trial. *European Urology, 71*(4), 534–542. doi:10.1016/j.eururo.2016.07.027

Virgo, K. S., Basch, E., Loblaw, D. A., Oliver, T. K., Rumble, R. B., Carducci, M. A., . . . Singer, E. A. (2017). Second-line hormonal therapy for men with chemotherapy-naive, castration-resistant prostate cancer: American Society of Clinical Oncology provisional clinical opinion. *Journal of Clinical Oncology*, 35(17), 1952–1964. doi:10.1200/JCO.2017.72.8030

Specific Articles for Gay Men

Capistrant, B. D., Torres, B., Merengwa, E., West, W. G., Mitteldorf, D., & Rosser, B. R. (2016). Caregiving and social support for gay and bisexual men with prostate cancer. *Psychooncology*, 25(11), 1329–1336. doi:10.1002/pon.4249

Chambers, S. K., Chung, E., Wittert, G., & Hyde, M. K. (2017). Erectile dysfunction, masculinity, and psychosocial outcomes: A review of the experiences of men after prostate cancer treatment. *Translational Andrology and Urology*, 6(1), 60–68. doi:10.21037/tau.2016.08.12

Dowsett, G. W., Lyons, A., Duncan, D., & Wassersug, R. J. (2014). Flexibility in men's sexual practices in response to iatrogenic erectile dysfunction after prostate cancer treatment. *Sexual Medicine*, 2(3), 115–120. doi:10.1002/sm2.32

Ussher, J. M., Perz, J., Kellett, A., Chambers, S., Latini, D., Davis, I. D., . . . Williams, S. (2016). Health-related quality of life, psychological distress, and sexual changes following prostate cancer: A comparison of gay and bisexual men with heterosexual men. *Journal of Sexual Medicine*, 13(3), 425–434. doi:10.1016/j.jsxm.2015.12.026

Ussher, J. M., Perz, J., & Simon Rosser, B. R. (Eds.). (2018). *Gay and bisexual men living with prostate cancer: From diagnosis to recovery*. New York, NY: Harrington Park Press.

ACKNOWLEDGMENTS

This book would not have been possible without the contributions of the androgen deprivation therapy (ADT) Working Group, a collection of approximately 20 people, including PhDs, MDs, nurses, and students, who work with, and are dedicated to helping, prostate cancer patients recognize and manage the side effects of their treatments. The ADT Working Group was established a decade ago and has been instrumental in helping us research, write, field test, edit, and revise this book. The authors and many contributors to this book are a part of the ADT Working Group.

We would also like to acknowledge the following people for their contributions:

Kirsten Kukula was *the* definitive editor of the first edition of this book, before moving on to medical school. Erik Wibowo took over the task of editor for the second edition and acted as a Program Coordinator for our ADT Educational Program. Kirsten Kukula and Erik Wibowo not only edited multiple drafts of the manuscript, but undertook key literature searches that contributed materially to every chapter in the book. We thank them profusely for tightening our writing. Every page has profited from their clarity of thought and comprehensive overview of this project. Erik Wibowo took on the challenging task of helping with the final copy editing of both editions of the book. We thank them both for their technical help. There is one more person to thank—Ms. Carly Sears, who helped us with the final proofreading of the text for this edition of the book.

Daniel Santa Mina and Andrew Matthew contributed to the development and writing of the chapter on exercise. Special thanks to Nicole Culos-Reed for additional input on the chapter on exercise. Andrew Matthew also provided feedback and editorial revisions on the first edition of the book.

Andrew Matthew and Kristen Currie contributed to the chapter on healthy eating. Cheri Van Patten extensively updated that chapter for the second edition and adapted its content for our U.S. audience.

Deborah McLeod is a founding member and driving force of the ADT Working Group.

Several physicians, who treat prostate cancer patients on ADT, offered critical review of the book, including Paul Abel, Shabbir Alibhai, Peter Black, Stacy Elliott, Dean Ruether, Kishore Visvanathan, and Derek Wilke.

The inclusion in this second edition of information specifically for gay and bisexual men was enriched by Richard Wassersug's collaboration with Tsz Kin (Bernard) Lee in Vancouver, British Columbia, and Gary Dowsett in Melbourne, Australia. Richard also thanks S. Larry Goldenberg for his commitment to developing supportive care resources for prostate cancer patients and their families in Vancouver. The Australian Research Centre in Sex, Health and Society provides Richard a research home in the southern hemisphere, and colleagues down under that share his interests in helping prostate cancer patients recover from the side effects of their cancer treatments.

The ADT Working Group has received financial support from a variety of sources.

The initial meeting of the group in 2008 was supported by grants from the Nova Scotia Health Research Foundation, the Dalhousie Cancer Research Program (now the Beatrice Hunter Cancer Research Institute), and a private donation from Lori Wood, MD.

Development and assessment of this book was supported by a grant from the Canadian Institutes of Health Research (Richard Wassersug and John Robinson, coprincipal investigators). Lauren Walker's dissertation research, which field-tested a draft of the first edition of the book, was supported by scholarships from the Social Sciences and Humanities Council of Canada, and Alberta Innovates–Health Solutions, as well as a Canadian Male Sexual Health Council Grant (John Robinson, Principal Investigator). Linette Lawlor, a summer student working with Lauren Walker and John Robinson, was funded by the Program for Undergraduate Research Experience, University of Calgary, to help her with the second revision.

We are pleased to acknowledge, in alphabetical order, the pharmaceutical companies that manufacture and market medications used in treating prostate cancer and have supported this work. We extend special thanks to Peter

Black for bringing this project to the attention of all those companies. Their broad support attests to the companies' commitment to meet the needs of prostate cancer patients dealing with the consequences of ADT.

AbbVie
Amgen
AstellasPharmaCanada, Inc.
AstraZeneca Canada, Inc.
Ferring, Inc.
Johnson & Johnson Shared Services (Janssen Biotech, Inc.)
Sanofi Canada

Several institutions deserve special mention for the long-term support that they have provided to the ADT Working Group:

- Dalhousie University, Capital Health, and the Nova Scotia Cancer Centre in Halifax, Nova Scotia
- Tom Baker Cancer Centre, University of Calgary, and Prostate Cancer Center in Calgary, Alberta
- Vancouver General Hospital, Vancouver Prostate Centre, British Columbia Cancer Agency, and the University of British Columbia in Vancouver, British Columbia
- Princess Margaret Cancer Center in Toronto, Ontario

INDEX

abdominal breathing, for hot flashes, 20–21
abiraterone (Zytiga), 3, 8, 27
Academy of Nutrition and Dietetics, 71
activities
   action plan, 34–35, 54–55, 99–100, 130–132, 142–143, 150–151, 162
   beliefs awareness (sexuality), 128–129, 168
   goal setting and confidence, 35–36, 55–57, 81, 100–101, 132, 143–144, 151–152, 163
   matching meaning and change using self-statements (exercise), 52
   mindfulness exercise, 93–94
   progressive muscle relaxation, 91–93
   pros/cons table, 33–34, 49, 50, 80, 98–99, 129–130, 141–142, 149–150, 161
   screening for emotional distress, 87–89, 166–167
   side effects self-assessment, 36–38, 164–165
acupuncture, 16
acute kidney failure, 32
acute myocardial infarction, 27
ADT. *See* androgen deprivation therapy
ADT2, 3
ADT3, 9
aerobic exercise, 43, 44–46
   high-intensity, 46
affection, 141
alcohol, 23
alpha-linolenic acid (omega-3; ALA), 65, 71–72
alprostadil (Caverject, Edex, Prostin VR), 124
Anandron (nilutamide), 4

androgen deprivation therapy (ADT)
   definition of, 1–2
   duration of, 10
   future of, 8–9
   impact on committed relationships, 137–146
   intermittent, 11, 12
   intimate relationships and, 105–135
   length of effectiveness of, 11–12
   lowers libido, 105
   origins of, 6–8
   overview of, 2–4
   pharmacological approach, 6
   psychological effects of, 156
   psychological well-being and, 85–102
   sexuality and, 105–135
   short-term, 10
   side effects of, 1, 15–39, 41, 43, 63
   surgical castration, 7
   use of PSA test with, 11–12
androgens, 1
   high-fat diet and, 65
anemia, 27–28
Aneros, 119
anger, 87
animal protein, 66
antiandrogens, 2
antidepressants, 18–19
antioxidants, 78, 79
anxiety, 85, 86, 90–91
asanas, 48
atorvastatin (Lipitor), 26
Avodart (dutasteride), 9

balance exercises, 43
beliefs awareness, 128–129, 168
benign prostatic hypertrophy (BPH), 9
bicalutamide (Casodex), 4
bimix, 124
biochemical failure, 11
biochemical relapse, 11
bisphosphonates, 23–24
blood clots, 18
blood pressure, 26, 47
blood sugar, 26, 90
blood thinners, 125
BMD. *See* bone mineral density
BMI. *See* body mass index
body fat percentage, 69
body hair loss, 31
body mass index (BMI), 69–70, 156
body odor, 32
bone density exam, 23
bone health, 47–48
bone mineral density (BMD), 23
bone weakening, 22–24
BPH. *See* benign prostatic hypertrophy
brain games, 97
breast cancer, 18, 29
breast enlargement, 28
breast irradiation, 29
breast reduction surgery, 29–30
breathing, during exercise, 43, 45, 47
buserelin (Suprefact), 4

CAB. *See* combined androgen blockade
caffeine, 23
calcium, 23, 76–78
calorie needs, 70–71
cancer diagnosis, 85
canola oil, 73
carbohydrates, 68–69
cardio training, 44
cardiovascular risk, 25–27, 43, 63
Casodex (bicalutamide), 4
castration, 6, 7
castration-resistant prostate cancer (CRPC), 6, 18
Caverject (alprostadil/prostaglandin E1), 124
chemotherapy, 8, 44
chronic illness, 2
Cialis (tadalafil), 123
clitoris, 118
cognitive behavioral therapy, 20
cognitive function, 86, 96–98
combined androgen blockade (CAB), 3

committed relationships, 137–146. *See also* noncommitted relationships
  activities for, 141–145
  essentials, 144
  for gay men, 148–149
  potential changes in, 138–141
complex carbohydrates, 68
confidence, 35–36, 55–57, 81, 100–101, 132, 143–144, 151–152, 163
coping style, differences in, 139
counseling, 91
  for hot flashes, 20
Crestor (rosuvastatin), 26
CRPC. *See* castration-resistant prostate cancer

dairy products, 66, 67
dating, 108–111
  being open and honest, 109–110
  new relationships and, 110–111
degarelix (Firmagon), 4, 5
denial, 96
denosumab (Xgeva), 24
Depo-Provera (medroxyprogesterone), 19
depression, 33, 85, 86, 89–90
DES. *See* diethylstilbestrol
Deuce, 120
DEXA. *See* dual-energy x-ray absorptiometry
DHT. *See* dihydrotestosterone
diabetes, 25, 43, 63, 90
Dietary Reference Intakes, 70, 75
diethylstilbestrol (DES), 3, 6
dihydrotestosterone (DHT), 1, 9
dildos, 119, 120
disaccharides, 68
docosahexaenoic acid (DHA), 71
drug chart, 158
dual-energy x-ray absorptiometry (DEXA), 23
dutasteride (Avodart), 9

eating healthy. *See* nutrition
ED. *See* erectile dysfunction
Edex (alprostadil/prostaglandin E1), 124
Effexor (venlafaxine), 18, 19
eicosapentaenoic acid (EPA), 71
ejaculation, 123
  orgasms without, 116–117
Eligard (leuprolide), 4, 6
ellagic acid, 78
emotional changes, 85, 101, 102, 156
emotional distress, screening for, 87–89, 166–167

emotional expression, 87, 96
emotional lability, 85
enzalutamide (Xtandi), 3, 27
erectile assistive aids, 122–128
    inflatable penile prosthesis, 125–126
    injections
        alprostadil, 124
        bimix, 124
        Caverject, 124
        Edex, 124
        prostaglandin E1, 124
        Prostin VR, 124
        trimix, 124
    intraurethral suppositories, 124–125
    oral medications
        Cialis, 123
        Levitra, 123
        phosphodiesterase-5 inhibitors, 123
        sildenafil, 123
        Staxyn, 123
        vardenafil, 123
        Viagra, 123
    vacuum pump, 125
erectile difficulties, 148
erectile dysfunction (ED), 30, 31, 108, 147
    treatments for, 121–122
erotic material, 116
estradiol, 3, 17–19, 98
estrogens, 3, 17–18
Eulexin (flutamide), 4
exercise, 24–27, 41–60
    aches and pains, 59
    action plan, 54–55
    in ADT context, 43
    aerobic, 43–46
    balance, 43
    barriers to, 49, 58–59
    benefits of, 41, 48, 96
    bone health, 47–48
    breathing during, 43, 45, 47
    comfortable clothing, 42
    essentials, 59–60
    goal setting, 55–57
    intensity of, 43–45
    making decision to, 49
    motivation for, 57–58
    preparation for, 53–54
    pro/cons table, 49, 50
    protective equipment, 42
    regular, 41
    resistance training, 43, 46–47
    safety, 42, 43, 46
    SMART goals, 51–52
    stretching, 43, 44, 49
    warm-up, 43–44
    water consumption, 42
    weight-bearing, 43, 48
    willpower, 59
    winding down, 49
external penile prosthesis, 120

fatigue, 27–28, 41, 58–59, 94–95
fats, 64–66
fiber, 68
finasteride (Proscar), 9
Firmagon (degarelix), 4, 5
fish, 66–67, 75
"flare," 5
fluoxetine (Prozac), 19, 20
flutamide (Eulexin), 4
food. *See also* nutrition
    calcium in, 76–78
    fresh, 64
    labels, 64
    processed, 64
    soy, 73–74
foreplay, 113, 117

gabapentin (Neurontin), 19, 20
gay men, 113–114
gay relationships
    committed relationship, 148–149
    essentials, 152–153
    noncommitted relationships, 148
    pros/cons table, 149–150
    sexual changes, 147
Generalized Anxiety Disorder 7-Item (GAD-7) Scale, 167
genital shrinkage, 30–31
GnRH agonists. *See* gonadotropin-releasing hormone agonists
GnRH antagonists. *See* gonadotropin-releasing hormone antagonists
goal setting, 35–36, 51, 52, 55–57, 81, 100–101, 132, 143–144, 151–152, 163
gonadotropin-releasing hormone (GnRH) agonists, 2
gonadotropin-releasing hormone (GnRH) antagonists, 2
goserelin (Zoladex), 4
grief, 85, 95–96
gynecomastia, 28–29

hair loss, 31
health, maintenance of, 155–156
healthy eating. *See* nutrition

heart attack, 27
hemoglobin, 28
high-density lipoproteins, 26
high-dose estradiol, 18
high-intensity aerobic exercise, 46
high-intensity interval training (HIIT), 46
HIIT. *See* high-intensity interval training
hip fractures, 22
hip pain, 24
hormone replacement therapy, 17
"hormone sensitive," 6
hormone therapy, 7
hot flashes (flushes), 15–22, 27
   abdominal breathing for, 20–21
   counseling for, 20
   diary for, 21–22, 160
   medications for, 17–20
   symptoms of, 15–16
   treatment for, 16, 18
hypothalamus, 5

immune system, 32
inflatable penile prosthesis (IPP), 125–126
injections, for erectile dysfunction, 124
insulin resistance, 90
intermittent hormonal therapy, 10
intimacy
   initiation of, 112
   maintaining, 137–138
   making time for, 108
   nonphysical, 106–107
intimate relationships, 105–135. *See also* sexuality
   date nights and, 108
   essentials, 133
   impact of ADT on, 137–146
   loss of libido and, 105–106
   nonsexual intimacy in, 106–108
   suggestions for enjoying sensual pleasure in, 112–116
intraurethral suppositories, 124–125. *See also* MUSE: Medicated Urethral System for Erection
iron deficiency, 28
isoflavones, 73, 78
Istubal (tamoxifen), 29

joint pain, 31, 32, 42

kidney disease, 32
kidney stones, 76

lapses, 57
legumes, 67
leuprolide (Lupron, Eligard), 4, 6
Levitra (vardenafil), 123
LHRH agonists. *See* luteinizing hormone-releasing hormone agonists
LHRH antagonists. *See* luteinizing hormone-releasing hormone antagonists
libido, 105–106, 112, 133, 140, 144, 147
lifestyle changes, 79
linoleic acid (omega-6; LA), 65, 72–73
Lipitor (atorvastatin), 26
long-term relationship, 147, 148
lubricants, 126–127
Lupron (leuprolide), 4, 6
luteinizing hormone-releasing hormone (LHRH) agonists, 2, 4–6, 15, 28, 31
luteinizing hormone-releasing hormone (LHRH) antagonists, 2, 4–6, 15, 31
lycopene, 79–80

MAB. *See* maximum androgen blockade
masculinity, 87, 95
mastalgia, 28
masturbation, 126
maximum androgen blockade (MAB), 3
medications
   chart, 158
   for erectile dysfunction, 123
   for hot flashes, 17–20
   for mental decline, 98
   types of, 2–4
medroxyprogesterone (Provera/Depo-Provera), 19, 20
megestrol (Megace), 19, 20
memory, 97
menopause, 16, 17
metabolic syndrome, 25–27
metastases, 5
metastatic disease, 5, 8, 11
metformin, 25, 26
milk, 67, 75
mind–body practice, 48–49
mindful awareness, 115
mindfulness meditation, 115
miso, 73
moderate-to-vigorous exercise, 45–46
monosaccharides, 68
monounsaturated fats, 65
mood swings, 85
motivation to exercise, 57–58
multitasking, 97
muscle loss, 24–25, 43, 46, 63
muscle pain, 32
muscle soreness, 42
MUSE: Medicated Urethral System for Erection, 124

natto, 73
Neurontin (gabapentin), 19, 20
night sweats, 16, 27
Nilandron (nilutamide), 4
nilutamide (Nilandron, Anandron), 4
nitroglycerin, 123
Nolvadex (tamoxifen), 29
noncommitted relationships, 148. *See also* committed relationships
non-insertive sex, Deuce, 120
nutrition, 63–82
   action plan, 81
   BMI, 69
   calcium, 76–78
   carbohydrates, 68–69
   essentials, 82
   estimating nutritional needs, 70–71
   fats, 64–66
   food labels and, 64
   goal setting and confidence, 81
   omega-3 fatty acids, 71–72
   omega-6 fatty acids, 72–73
   phytonutrients, 78
   pros/cons of changing, 80
   protein, 66–68
   recommendations, 64, 66, 68, 69, 72–73, 77
   soy, 73–74
   vitamin D, 74–75

obesity, 65
   sarcopenic, 25
olive oil, 73
omega-3 fatty acids, 65, 71–72
omega-6 fatty acids, 72–73
ONJ. *See* osteonecrosis of the jaw
oral sex, 117, 118, 127
orchiectomy, 6–7, 27
orgasm, 113, 114, 118
   without ejaculation, 116–117
osteonecrosis of the jaw (ONJ), 23–24
osteopenia, 22
osteoporosis, 22, 24, 76

paced respiration, for hot flashes, 20
papaverine, 124
paroxetine (Paxil), 19, 20
partially hydrogenated oils, 65
Patient Health Questionnaire-9 (PHQ-9), 166
Paxil (paroxetine), 19, 20
pedometers, 46
penetrative sex, 120
penile shrinkage, 30–31
penile sleeve, 120

Percent Daily Value (%DV), 64
periodontal disease, 32
petroleum-based lubricants, 127
phentolamine, 124
phosphodiesterase-5 inhibitors (PDE5i), 123
physical side effects, 15–39
   anemia, 27–28
   body hair loss, 31
   bone weakening, 22–24
   breast enlargement, 28
   cardiovascular risk, 25–27, 43
   diabetes, 25, 43
   erectile dysfunction, 121, 123
   essentials about, 38
   fatigue, 27–28
   genital shrinkage, 30–31
   hot flashes, 15–22, 27
   metabolic syndrome, 25–27
   muscle loss, 24–25, 43, 46, 63
   questionnaire, 164–165
   self-assessment of, 36–38
   weight gain, 24–25, 41, 63
phytonutrients, 78
pituitary gland, 4–5
plant protein, 67–68
pneumonia, 32
polyphenols, 78
polysaccharides, 68
polyunsaturated fats, 65
pomegranate, 78
pornography, 116
pranayama, 48
processed food, 64
progesterone, 19
progressive muscle relaxation, 91–93
Proscar (finasteride), 9
prostaglandin E1 (Caverject, Edex, Prostin VR), 124
prostate cancer, 30, 155
   androgen synthesis blocker drugs, 4
   antiandrogen drugs for, 4
   chemotherapy for, 8
   as chronic illness, 2
   LHRH drugs, 4
   treatment, 148
prostate-specific antigen (PSA), 6, 10–12
Prostin VR (alprostadil/prostaglandin E1), 124
protein, 66–68
Provera (medroxyprogesterone), 19, 20
Prozac (fluoxetine), 19, 20
PSA. *See* prostate-specific antigen
PSA chart, 159
PSA test, 11–12, 18, 86

Index

psychological well-being, 85–102
  activities for, 100–101
  anxiety, 90–91
  cognition, 96–98
  depression, 90
  emotional distress, 86
  emotional expression, 87, 96
  essentials of, 101
  fatigue, 94–95
  grief, 95–96
  progressive muscle relaxation, 91–93
  self-assessment, 87–89
psychotherapy, 91
punicalagin, 78

qualified exercise professional (QEP)
  exercise safety, 42–44, 59
  qualification and training, 42

radiation therapy, 10, 44
Rating of Perceived Exertion (RPE) Scale, 44
red meat, 66
relapses, 57
relaxation technique, 20
resistance training, 43, 46–47
rewards, 57–58
rosuvastatin (Crestor), 26

sarcopenia, 25
saturated fats, 65
second-line hormonal therapies, 12
selective estrogen-receptor modulator (SERM), 29
selective serotonin reuptake inhibitors (SSRIs), 18, 19
self-assessment
  for emotional distress, 87–89
  side effects, 164–165
self-doubt, 140–141
self-identity, 95
self-image, 30
self-statements, 52
serotonin norepinephrine reuptake inhibitors (SNRIs), 18
sex drive, 137
sex toys. *See* sexual aids and sex toys
sexual
  activities, 112–113
  appetite, 115–116
  changes, 147
  function, 147
  intercourse, 107, 117
  issues, 148
  relationship, 111–112
  touch, decreased responsiveness to, 114

sexual aids and sex toys
  Aneros, 119
  Cobra Libre, 119
  for masturbation, 126, 127
  Pulse, 119
  Viberect, 119
  vibrators, 119, 121
  Wahl vibrator, 119
sexual devices to permit insertive sex without erections
  external penile prosthesis, 120
  penile sleeve, 120
  SpareParts, 120
  strap-on dildo, 120
sexuality, 95, 105–135, 156. *See also* intimate relationships
  activities, 128–132
  beliefs about, 128–129
  beyond intercourse, 117–118
  brain, 111
  developing new sexual practices, 127–128
  erectile dysfunction, 121–126
  essentials, 133
  loss of libido, 105–106
  mindfulness exercise, 93–94
  oral sex, 117–118, 127
  orgasm, 113, 114
  pros/cons table, 129–130
  questions for couples, 134
  responsiveness, 114
  role of, 111
  sex toys, 118–121, 126, 127
  suggestions for, 112–116
side effects. *See* physical side effects
sildenafil (Viagra), 123
silicone lubricants, 127
simple carbohydrates, 68
sleep, night sweats and, 16, 27
SMART goals, 51–52
smoking, 23
SNRIs. *See* serotonin norepinephrine reuptake inhibitors
social support, 58
solo masturbation, 126
soy, 16, 73–74
soy beverages, 73
soy powder, 74
soy sauce, 74
SpareParts, 120
spontaneous sex, 147
SSRIs. *See* selective serotonin reuptake inhibitors
stair climbing, 45
starches, 68
statins, 26

Staxyn (vardenafil), 123
staying healthy, 155–156
strap-on dildo, 120
strength training, 46–47
stress, 85
   management, 99
stretching, 43, 44, 49
sugars, 68
sunlight, 74
supplements, 23, 33, 78
   iron, 28
   omega-3, 71–72
Suprefact (buserelin), 4
surgical castration, 7
sweating, 16

TAB. *See* total androgen blockade
tadalafil (Cialis), 123
tai chi, 48–49
talk test, 45
tamari, 74
tamoxifen (Nolvadex, Istubal, Valodex), 29
tearfulness, 87
tempeh, 73
testicles, 4
   shrinkage of, 30
testosterone, 1, 9, 15, 123
   cognition, 96
   depression, 90
   effects of, 1
   high-fat diet, 65
   production, 5, 6
   sex drive, 111
   sexual responsiveness, 114
textured vegetable protein (TVP), 73
tofu, 73
total androgen blockade (TAB), 3
trans fats, 65
transdermal, 17, 24

Trelstar (triptorelin), 4
triglycerides, 26
trimix, 124
triple blockade, 9
triptorelin (Trelstar), 4

unsaturated fats, 65
urination, 30
U.S. Department of Agriculture, 71

vacuum erection device (VED), 31, 125
Valodex (tamoxifen), 29
vardenafil (Levitra, Staxyn), 123
VED. *See* vacuum erection device
venlafaxine (Effexor), 18, 19
Viagra (sildenafil), 123
Viberect, 119
vibrators, 119, 121
vitamin D, 23, 74–75

Wahl vibrator, 119
waist circumference, 26, 70
waist-to-hip ratio, 69
walking, 44, 45, 48
warfarin, 125
warm-up exercises, 43–44
water-based lubricants, 127
weight gain, 24–25, 41, 63
weight lifting, 46–47
weight-bearing exercises, 43, 48
willpower, 59

Xgeva (denosumab), 24

yoga, 48–49

Zoladex (goserelin), 4
Zytiga (abiraterone), 3, 8, 27

ABOUT THE AUTHORS

Richard J. Wassersug, PhD, is a research scientist who earned his doctoral degree in evolutionary biology from the University of Chicago. He then spent most of his career studying the biology of amphibians and teaching anatomy in the medical school at Dalhousie University in Halifax, Nova Scotia. At the age of 52, he was diagnosed with prostate cancer and has received multiple treatments for the disease. After beginning androgen deprivation therapy, he redirected his research to study the psychology of androgen deprivation in various populations. Richard now holds the title of Honorary Professor at the University of British Columbia, Vancouver, Canada, and Adjunct Professor in the Australian Research Centre in Sex, Health and Society, La Trobe University, Melbourne, Australia.

Lauren M. Walker, PhD, R Psych, is an adjunct assistant professor in the Department of Oncology's Division of Psychosocial Oncology at the University of Calgary's Cumming School of Medicine. She is a registered clinical psychologist in the province of Alberta, and works clinically in the Department of Psychosocial Resources at the Tom Baker Cancer Centre. She completed a clinical fellowship in 2015, specializing in oncology and sexuality. Her passion is in helping cancer patients adapt to sexual changes after cancer treatment. She received her doctorate in clinical psychology in 2013 from the University of Calgary's Clinical Psychology Program. There she completed her dissertation research evaluating a patient education initiative for preparing prostate cancer patients (and their partners) starting androgen deprivation therapy. Dr. Walker established the University of Calgary's Oncology Sexual Health Lab and maintains an active research program. She was recently recognized with the 2017 President's New Researcher Award from the Canadian Psychological Association and the 2016 Young Investigator Award for Excellence in Research from the Department of Oncology at the University of Calgary. She is an active researcher, who has contributed several key articles to the scientific literature on the psychosocial adaptation to androgen deprivation therapy, sexual adaptation after prostate cancer treatment, and interventions for women's sexual health after cancer treatments.

John W. Robinson, PhD, R Psych, has been a clinical psychologist and a member of the Genitourinary Gynaecological Cancer Programs at the Tom Baker Cancer Centre in Calgary, Alberta, since 1986. He concurrently provides clinical service and creates and evaluates new ways to ease the psychological burden of cancer on not just patients but also their loved ones. He has appointments in both oncology and clinical psychology at the University of Calgary, where he teaches and carries on an active research program.

CONTRIBUTORS

Kristen L. Currie, MA, CCRP, graduated in 2002 from Queen's University in Kingston, Ontario, with concurrent degrees in life science and physical and health education. She then completed a master's degree in 2005 in kinesiology (health psychology) at York University in Toronto, Ontario. In her previous role as manager of the Prostate Cancer Rehabilitation Clinic at Princess Margaret Cancer Centre in Toronto, she researched nutrition behavior of men at risk of onset or recurrence of prostate cancer. Kristen currently works for Cancer Care Ontario as a senior analyst in the Quality Management Partnership.

Kirsten C. Kukula, BSc, MD, holds two degrees from Dalhousie University. In 2011, she completed a Bachelor of Science Co-op, with combined honors in biology, sociology, and social anthropology. In 2018, she received her Doctor of Medicine. Her areas of professional interest include the social determinants of health, palliative care, sexuality, and rural/remote medicine.

Linette Lawlor-Savage, MSc, is completing doctoral studies in clinical psychology at the University of Calgary. Her primary interest areas are neuropsychology and psychosocial oncology. Her current research utilizes behavioral and neuroimaging methods to investigate cognitive functioning (e.g., loss and recovery of abilities such as memory, thinking speed, and decision making) in healthy aging adults and in cancer survivors.

Andrew Matthew, PhD, C Psych, is a senior staff psychologist at the Princess Margaret Cancer Hospital in Toronto, Ontario, where he is a clinician–investigator in the Department of Surgery, Division of Urology, and a member of the Department of Psychosocial Oncology and Palliative Care. He is also an assistant professor in the Faculty of Medicine, University of Toronto, Departments of Surgery and Psychiatry.

Deborah McLeod, RN, PhD, is a clinician scientist in nursing with the Queen Elizabeth II Cancer Care Program in Halifax, Nova Scotia, where she is a clinical member of a psychosocial oncology team providing individual, couples, and family therapy. She holds academic appointments at Dalhousie University (adjunct) and the University of Calgary (adjunct associate professor) and consults on web-based education and therapeutic interventions.

Daniel Santa Mina, CEP, PhD, is an assistant professor at the University of Toronto in the Faculty of Kinesiology and Physical Education and the Faculty of Medicine in the Department of Surgery. Dr. Santa Mina is also a scientist in the Cancer Rehabilitation and Survivorship Program at the Princess Margaret Cancer Centre where he is the lead for Exercise Programming. Dr. Santa Mina completed his PhD in kinesiology at York University and postdoctoral fellowship in the Department of Surgical Oncology at the Princess Margaret Cancer Centre. He is a registered kinesiologist and certified exercise physiologist with advanced training in oncology. Dr. Santa Mina's main areas of clinical-research focus are on the physiological, functional, and psychosocial effects of exercise for cancer survivors, and in particular, men with prostate cancer. Dr. Santa Mina is also heavily involved in strategies for bringing exercise into standard cancer care.

Cheri Van Patten, RD, MSc, is a registered dietitian with over 22 years of combined clinical and research experience in prostate cancer at the British Columbia Cancer Agency in Vancouver. Her areas of expertise and publications have included diet, body weight, obesity, exercise, and dietary supplements, and their impact on quality of life and risk of recurrence in cancer survivors.

Erik Wibowo, PhD, is a lecturer in the Department of Anatomy at the University of Otago. He completed his PhD at Dalhousie University where he conducted studies in animal models on how androgen deprivation with and without estradiol influences sleep and sexual behaviors. Following his doctoral studies, he did his postdoctoral training at the Vancouver Prostate Centre where he managed an educational program for patients on androgen deprivation therapy (ADT) and their partners. His area of research focuses on how ADT side effects can be alleviated.

CPSIA information can be obtained
at www.ICGtesting.com
Printed in the USA
LVHW102300150419
614311LV00009B/142/P